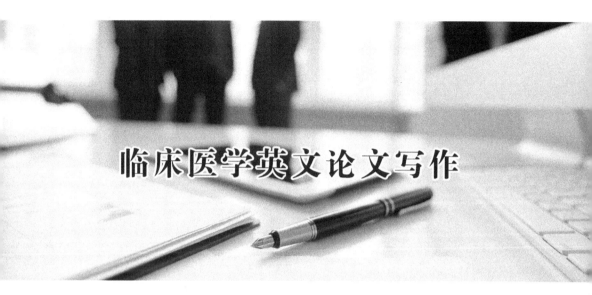

临床医学英文论文写作

● 编著／廖联明　黄　静

U0380028

东南大学出版社
SOUTHEAST UNIVERSITY PRESS
·南京·

图书在版编目(CIP)数据

临床医学英文论文写作 / 廖联明,黄静编著. — 南京 : 东南大学出版社,2023.9(2024.8 重印)

ISBN 978 - 7 - 5766 - 0849 - 6

Ⅰ. ①临… Ⅱ. ①廖… ②黄… Ⅲ. ①医学—英语论文—写作 Ⅳ. ①R

中国国家版本馆 CIP 数据核字(2023)第 159219 号

责任编辑:陈潇潇 责任校对:周 菊 封面设计:王 玥 责任印制:周荣虎

临床医学英文论文写作
LINCHUANG YIXUE YINGWEN LUNWEN XIEZUO

编 著	廖联明 黄 静	
出版发行	东南大学出版社	
出 版 人	白云飞	
社 址	南京四牌楼 2 号 邮编:210096	
网 址	http://www.seupress.com	
电子邮件	press@seupress.com	
经 销	全国各地新华书店	
印 刷	广东虎彩云印刷有限公司	
开 本	700 mm×1 000 mm 1/16	
印 张	13.75	
字 数	200 千字	
版 次	2023 年 9 月第 1 版	
印 次	2024 年 8 月第 3 次印刷	
书 号	ISBN 978 - 7 - 5766 - 0849 - 6	
定 价	52.00 元	

* 本社图书若有印装质量问题,请直接与营销部调换。电话(传真):025 - 83791830。

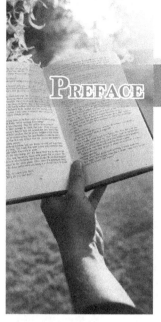

PREFACE 前言 •••

临床医学英文论文写作
A Guide to Writing Medical Papers in English

学者们都知道"要么出版，要么灭亡"（Publish or perish）：发表原创研究，否则你的学术地位将受到影响，甚至失去职位。

"Publish or perish"这个短语可以追溯到1942年，当时社会学家洛根·威尔逊（Logan Wilson）在一本研究学者职业生涯的书中使用了它。他将"Publish or perish"的信条描述为"强加在学术团体身上的普遍实用主义（prevailing pragmatism forced upon the academic group）"。80多年过去了，今天的学者仍有这种感觉。对于在"Publish or perish"信条下生存的人来说，这是一种压力很大的工作方式。甚至有人拿这句话和莎士比亚的名句"To be or not to be, that is a question."做对比，提出了"To publish or perish, that is a question."，可见论文发表的重要性。

为什么要发表文章？

首先，也是最重要的是，发表文章的目的是与国际科学界分享研究成果。这是积累知识不可或缺的一步。它不仅可以帮助同行在你的研究基础上进一步深入，避免重复性工作，而且通过发表文章还可以接受同行的批评、反馈，包括该领域最杰出的专家的建议和意见，有助于不断提高研究质量，纠正工作中尚未被发现的错误、缺陷和偏差。如果研究结果无法传达给其他人，那么研究就没有什么价值。研究项目只有在研究文章发表并被他人阅读、理解和相信后才能算最终完成。这是发表论文的初衷。

其次，是一个社会责任。由于社会直接或间接资助了研究，因此它应该有机会看到结果并评估研究人员的表现。

再次，临床研究的发表能够产生临床和社会影响。例如，可以帮助临床医生提高医疗质量、完善治疗指南和改善患者健康，或者促进公共卫生干预。

最后，科学出版是成功的学术生涯的重要组成部分，也是申请新的研究资金的重要手段。学术界必须发表研究成果才能体现学术性。在大多学术机构这是一项关键的绩效指标。著作的多少可以用来确定一位学者在一个机构的价值，也可以决定谁将获得晋升。

可以想象，出版论文的压力非常大。不幸的是，发表论文正在变得越来越困难，部分原因是全世界的学者数量在增加，学术机构对学者的要求也在提高。

不管你喜不喜欢，"Publish or perish"是当今学术界的现实。在这样一个饱和的，有时甚至是残酷的体系中，要不通过竞争脱颖而出，要不被淘汰。既然"Publish or perish"制度不可能在短期内消失，我们能够做的只能是运用各种途径，增加发表论文的机会。

即使很好地完成了一项研究，如果文章写得不好，也无法很好地体现研究的价值。写好论文并非易事。除了在写作过程中保持良好的状态外，掌握一些写作技巧可以使论文撰写更有效。

当时还是哈佛大学研究生的 Anne Margaret Lee 在《Nature》写过一个短文《Writer's block》。她在文中写道[1]：

无论是对于科学的进步，对于个人的职业生涯，还是对于一个有争议的理论，出版的重要性都是毋庸置疑的。虽然我有时想忽略它的价值，但我做不到"。（*Whether for the advancement of science, of one's career or of a controversial theory, the importance of publishing remains incontrovertible. Although I'd sometimes like to ignore its significance, I can't.*）

尤其是现在，我第一次面对写作的任务。数据就在那里。数据和我两年前第一次开始这个项目时想象的那样，构成了一个有趣的故事。但是把这个故事完整地展现出来并让科学界其他人都感兴趣是一个挑战。（*Especially now, when I find myself facing the task of writing my first paper. The data are nearly there. It's almost the interesting story I imagined it would be when I first began the project two years ago. But it's a challenge to put the story into a package that the rest of the scientific community will find interesting.*）

要做到这一点，我需要了解它在已有的科学知识中的重要性。我需要强调我的故事是多么的新奇和与众不同，以及为什么它值得发表。至少，我必须让素不相识的同行审稿专家相信，我的数据为整体的知识增添了一些重要的东西。（*To do that, I need to understand its place in the context of what has come before. I need to highlight how my story is new and different —and why it deserves to published. At the very least, I have to convince unknown peer reviewers that my data add something of importance to the collective knowledge.*）

我以前从未写过一篇论文，我想知道我是否能令人信服地做到这一点。可能是因为我对做不到感到焦虑，所以我还没有开始写作。我想我日益增加的不应该是焦虑，应该是兴奋。（*Having never written a paper before, I wonder if I will be able to do this convincingly at all. It may be that my anxiety at not being able to do so is the reason I haven't started writing yet. And I wonder whether my increasing anxiety should be excitement instead.*）

不管有没有焦虑和不自信，我知道我必须开始写作。否则，我的工作将无法发表——这对任何雄心勃勃的研究者来说都是一场噩梦。（*Anxiety and doubts or not, I know that I have to start writing. Otherwise, my work will remain unpublished — a nightmare for any ambitious researcher.*）

所谓"Writer's block"（写作障碍）是一种抑郁的感觉，感觉写作是很痛苦的事。这种想法通常源于对失败的恐惧，导致内心焦虑，甚至无法开始。即使开始了看起来也像是一项永远无法完成的任务。当然，障碍存在于头脑中，可以通过训练和努力来克服它。最可怕的时刻总是在你开始之前，而真的开始之后事情只会变得更好。

困难摆在面前，而且没有退路。为了确保成功，我们要认识到，学术期刊只挑选高质量的研究。除了确保您的研究有价值之外，论文的条理必须清晰，用词必须准确。不要因为语法或拼写错误降低了审稿人的兴趣。严格按照目标杂志的要求排版。面对如此激烈的竞争，你不能因为忽视期刊的投稿指南或风格而被拒稿。

国际医学期刊编辑委员会（International Committee of Medical Journal Editors，ICMJE）为了促进医学期刊的作者、编辑以及审稿人的工作，促进准确、清晰、可重复、无偏倚的医学期刊论文的创作和传播，编写了"生物医学期刊投稿的统一要求"（Uniform Requirements for Manuscripts Submitted to Biomedical Journals，URM）。URM 首次发表于 1978 年，后期更名为"医学期刊学术研究的实施、报告、编辑与发表建议"（Recommendations for the Conduct，Reporting，Editing，and Publication of Scholarly Work in Medical Journals），这是很好的一个写作指南。但指南毕竟太浓缩。

对一些人来说，这可能是你第一次不得不写英语文章。英语不是我们的母语，但没人会为你在写作中遇到的问题而同情你。你们不仅要毕业，还要为未来的事业做好准备。几乎所有的高校和大医院都希望他们的职员能够用英语进行有效的书面和口头交流。

如果被拒稿了，不要放弃。改投其他期刊，接受编辑和审稿人的建议，并仔细修改。这个过程可能很艰难，但坚持不懈一定会有回报。

写作期间尽量避免任何干扰，如电话、微信和回复电子邮件。当你觉得进展顺利时，可以顺其自然，延长写作时间；没有思路的时候就停止写作。最后一点是在达到中期和最终目标时奖励自己！

希望这本书可以帮助你实现这个目标。

本书是在福建医科大学研究生教学过程中不断完善下完成的。感谢在写作过程中福建医科大学附属协和医院中心实验室的大力支持！

参考文献

[1] Lee A. Writer's block. Nature，2005，434(7031)：418.

临床医学英文论文写作
A Guide to Writing Medical Papers in English

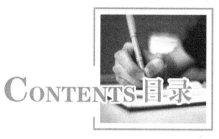

CONTENTS·目录

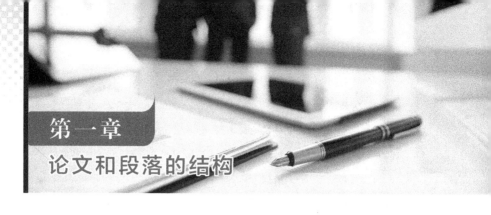

第一章
论文和段落的结构

　　原创性研究的论文（Original report），其正文通常分为引言（Introduction）、方法（Methods）、结果（Results）和讨论（Discussion）四个部分，即所谓的"IMRaD"结构。IMRaD 是"Introduction，Methods，Results，and Discussion"的首字母缩写。

第 1 节　论文格式的沿革

　　自 1665 年科学论文诞生以来，结构发生了重大变化[1]。早期的形式和风格没有标准化，主要以信件（Letter）和实验报告的形式为主。信件通常只有一位作者，以礼貌的方式写作，有时候会涉及好几个主题。实验报告则是描述性的，通常按时间顺序呈现。

　　19 世纪下半叶开始出现方法的描述，出现了现代论文的雏形：理论＋实验＋讨论（Theory-Experiment-Discussion）。20 世纪初，标准化的论文格式开始被出版界接受，文学风格的使用越来越少。从 20 世纪 60 年代开始，最具代表性的《英国医学杂志》（《British Medical Journal》，《BMJ》）、《柳叶刀》（《Lancet》）、《美国医学会杂志》（《Journal of American Medical Association》，《JAMA》）和《新英格兰医学杂志》（《New England Journal of Medicine》，《NEJM》）几乎完全采用现代格式，其他医学期刊也逐步效仿它们（表 1.1、图 1.1）。这种格式就是沿用到现在的 IMRaD 格式。这些历史悠久的杂志还少量保留了前期的"Letter"。有些论文在讨论后包括一小段的结论（Conclusion）。讨论也有叫"Comment"的。也有结果和讨论合并的短篇论文（Introduction，Materials and method，Results and discussion）。

表 1.1　论文格式的变迁

时间	变化
1665	科技论文出现
1600s—1700s	"Letter"和描述性研究格式并存
1800s 下半叶	增加方法部分
1900s(早期)	采用书信格式
1900s(下半叶)	IMRaD 格式开始出现
1950—1960	IMRaD 格式被部分杂志接受
1965 后	IMRaD 格式普及
1970	International Committee of Medical Journal Editors 出版指南
1980	IMRaD 格式完全主导

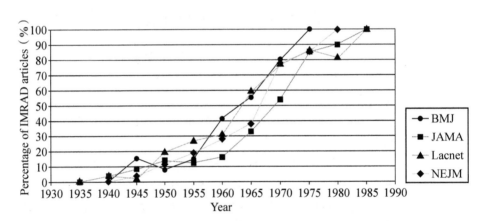

图 1.1　不同年代 IMRaD 格式在四大医学杂志的采用程度

第 2 节　如何开始写作

写作的顺序不必与文章各部分的顺序相同,可以先从自己认为最容易的部分开始以增强写作信心。一般来说引言和讨论部分是最难的,方法和结果比较容易。讨论部分的内容取决于论文中的发现,因此适合放最后写。建议按照这样的顺序写:

1. 先组织完整的"故事情节",即论文框架,特别是方法和结果部分。大家知道,科学界总是喜欢把文章说成一个故事,因此全部章节要形成一个符合逻辑和令人信服的故事。

2. 写完整的段落之前,使用几个主题词或一行文字说明每个段落的主要信息。

3. 创建空表格和草图并和主要作者讨论。

4. 收集与论文相关的主要参考文献,并将每篇文献需要的内容做好笔记,计划论文中需要引用的地方。

5. 在主题词的基础上,结合参考文献,构建段落。

6. 不断修改句子,直到整个段落读起来很顺。

7. 确认段落之间有过渡,段落之间读起来很顺。

8. 使用 Word 程序自带工具,初步确认没有语法和拼写错误。

在想如何开始之前,先想想在何时何地能够最平静、最有创造力、最富有成效地写论文。什么样的环境适合你?你最集中精力、最不分心的地方在哪里?一周中的哪一天、一天中的哪一个时间对写作最有成效?是不是需要采用休假时间写论文?

写作之前一定要构思好!第一作者以及论文的主要作者都必须就主要研究目标和主要结果达成一个清晰的共识。作者之间的讨论有助于写出一个清晰的故事。在写作早期选择目标期刊和目标受众也很重要。

第 3 节　稿件的构成

按照 International Committee of Medical Journal Editors 出版指南的推荐,投稿的时候一般按照以下顺序展开:

1. 标题页(Title page):包括标题、作者、单位(Affiliation)。

2. 摘要和关键词(Abstract and keywords)。

3. 正文(Text):前言、方法、结果和讨论。

4. 参考文献(References)。

5. 致谢(Acknowledgment)。

6. 利益冲突(Conflict of interest)。

7. 数据获取声明(Data sharing statements)。

8. 脚注(Footnotes)。

9. 图注(Figure legends),包括标题。

10. 表格(每个表单独一页)。

11. 图(每个图单独一页)。

12. 附录(Appendices)。

13. 网络补充材料(Online only supplementary materials)。

注意：每个部分都从新的一页开始。两页之间要用插入分页符的方法隔开，不能用回车键的方法分页。

第4节　标题页

标题页(Title page)是第一页，标题上方留2～3行空间。将其居中并采用粗体字体。

关于标题的大小写，有两种格式，即"Sentence case"（也称为"Down style"和"Reference style"）和"Title case"。常规的"Sentence case"只有第一个单词的首字母和专有名词大写。如：

➢ Forced enhancer-promoter rewiring to alter gene expression in animal models

在"Title case"中，第一个单词、最后一个单词和主要单词(Major word 或 Principal word)首字母大写，次要单词(Minor word)首字母小写。次要单词包括冠词(an、a 和 the)、连词(and、or 和 but)和介词(in、with 和 of)。如：

➢ Association of Preapproval Confirmatory Trial Initiation and Conversion to Traditional Approval or Withdrawal in the FDA Approval Pathway

不过，对于包含 4 个或以上字母的次要单词，如"with"，"between"和"from"，有些杂志要求首字母要大写。

复合名词的每个单词首字母都要大写，如"Self-Report"，不是"Self-report"。

有些杂志允许有副标题(Subtitle)，尤其是临床研究论文的标题往往通过副标题说明研究方法的类型。副标题一般采用冒号分开。副标题的首字母是大写还是小写，每个杂志不一样，如：

➢ Diagnosis and Treatment of Pulmonary Sarcoidosis：A Review

➢ Effect of Intra-arterial Alteplase vs Placebo Following Successful Thrombectomy on Functional Outcomes in Patients With Large Vessel Occlusion Acute Ischemic Stroke：The CHOICE Randomized Clinical Trial

➢ Recombinant human erythropoietin in transfusion-dependent anemic patients with multiple myeloma and non-Hodgkin lymphoma：a randomized multicenter study by the European Study Group of Erythropoietin(Epoetin Beta) Treatment in Multiple Myeloma and Non-Hodgkin's Lymphoma

作者行称为"byline"。如果有两位作者,作者之间使用"and";如果有三位或三位以上的作者,作者姓名之间加一个逗号,并在最后的作者姓名前使用"and"一词。但也有杂志不使用"and",如《JAMA》。有些杂志要求作者名字后标注学位,如《JAMA》。如果名字和学位之间有逗号,相应地,学位后面要用分号将每个作者分开,如:Mahnum Shahzad,BA;Huseyin Naci,MHS,PhD;Anita K. Wagner,PharmD,MPH,DrPH。因此一定要注意每个杂志的要求。

当不同的作者属于不同的单位时,在作者姓名后使用上标数字(有些杂志用符号)将姓名与相应的单位连接起来。如果所有作者都属于相同的单位,则不需要使用上标数字或符号,如:

➤ Stuart T. Fraser,[1] Joan Isern,[2] and Margaret H. Baron[3]

单位是完成该论文研究的机构,不一定是目前上班的地方。一般包括"department""college"和"university",城市和国家之间用逗号分隔,如:

➤ Department of Health Policy, London School of Economics and Political Science, London, United Kingdom

目前工作的单位如果和论文中的单位不一样,可以在脚注中注明。

研究合作组(Study group)名称也可作为署名。一般采用组名的缩写,避免太长,如:FOENIX-CCA2 Study Investigators,然后在附录中列出合作组的全部成员。在摘要或文章第一次出现合作组名字的时候,要标注,如:

➤ A complete list of the members of the XX Study Group appears in the "Appendix."

有时采用代表性的作者加合作组名称的方法,如:

➤ Ute Riedel, Axel Hinke, Stefanie Srock, Stefan Serke, Christian Peschel, and Bertold Emmerich, for the German Leukemia Study Group

在极少数情况下,研究合作组可能会作为唯一的作者显示。

共同第一作者用上标标注,如:

➤ * These authors contributed equally to this study.

或者用名字缩写,如:

➤ H. K. K. and M. D. L. contributed equally to this study.

通讯作者,包括多个通讯作者,也要用上标注明。

标头,即"Running heads",放在每一页页眉,这是早年纸质杂志留下来的风格,作用有二:一是审稿时方便找稿件,二是论文出版可以提醒读者文章的标题和方便翻阅杂志找到文章。单纯的网络版杂志一般不再采用这种形式。

左边的标头由作者的姓组成。一般来说如果有 3 位或更多作者，只显示第一位作者的姓和"et al"。当一篇文章只有两位作者时，一般使用"and"连接两位作者的姓。当只有一位作者时，只需使用该作者的姓即可。如：

➤ VAN KEMENADE et al

➤ VAN KEMENADE and LO-COCO

➤ LO-COCO

右边的标头是短标题（Short title）。短标题是论文标题的缩写版（如果标题已经很短，也可以作为短标题）。短标题也叫"Running title"。

一般短标题不超过 50 个字符（Character）。字符包括字母、空格（Space）和标点符号。比如"Running head"这个短语就有 11 个字母和一个空格，那么这个短语的总字符数是 12 个。短标题是一个意思完整并通顺的短语，因此不但要简短，还要明晰、扼要。好的短标题会给读者留下深刻印象。

为了尽可能减少字数，有些杂志允许在短标题中用缩写词，用"&"代替"and"。

如果论文曾经入选某个大会，一般要在标题页注明。有些杂志还要求在"Cover Letter"中也注明：

➤ Presented in abstract form at the 57th annual meeting of the American Society of Hematology, Orlando, FL.

有些杂志要求被接受的文章在修改稿的标题页注明"Submit""Accept"和"Publish"日期。

如果文章附有补充数据（如视频、电子表格），则也在标题页上注明："The online version of the article contains a data supplement"。

第 5 节　正　文

文章正文包括引言、方法、结果和讨论。这 4 个部分（Sections）大概的内容可以概括为 4 个"W"：

Introduction：Why did you start?

Methods：What did you do?

Results：What did you find?

Discussion：What does it all mean?

此外还可能包括致谢和/或附录。

Introduction、Methods、Results 和 Discussion 属于主标题（Main headings），即一级标题（First-level headings）。临床研究的论文方法部分的标题可以有："Materials and methods"，"Patients and methods"，"Participants and methods"或者"Patients，materials，and methods"。

副标题（Subheadings）应平行构建；每个部分可以有 2 个或以上副标题。一般来说第二级标题是单独的一行（与主标题一样），但第三级和第四级标题往往不单独一行，而是作为后续段落中的第一个短语，并用黑体体现，后加句号。标题中不引用参考文献。

致谢使用"Acknowledgments"或"Acknowledgment"。如果只有一个人或机构需要致谢，则用"Acknowledgment"。"Acknowledgment(s)"常常包括以下内容：

1. 和获得学位有关的研究声明

➢ A. B. C. and D. E. F. are PhD candidates at Any University and this work is submitted in partial fulfillment of the requirement for the PhD.

2. 纪念

➢ This work is in memory of XXX，who died while helping the authors with this article.

3. 基金支持

包括所有支持本研究的组织和个人。一般需要具体指定哪位作者获得了哪个支持，可通过插入括号中的名字首字母表示。如：

➢ This work was supported by grants from the Swiss National Science Foundation(81BS-52825)(B. U. M.) and the National Institutes of Health (grants CA41456 and CA72009)(D. G. T.).

4. 患者

➢ We especially thank the mothers who graciously agreed to volunteer for this study.

5. 未作为作者的个人的贡献

在介绍作者贡献（Contribution）时，有的杂志作者用全名，有的杂志有缩写，可以一段或分段介绍。

一段式介绍：

> DC reviewed the treatment records, carried out statistical analysis and drafted the manuscript. SW reviewed the treatment records and assisted in manuscript preparation. VL participated in the design of the study and assisted in the statistical analysis. JT assisted in data analysis and drafting the manuscript. All authors read and approved the final manuscript.

> Contributors：SS had the original idea for article, BD did the literature research, and both authors contributed to writing the article. SS managed the patient.

分段介绍：

> Conception and design：L. M. Schwartz, S. Woloshin, H. G. Welch.

> Analysis and interpretation of the data：L. M. Schwartz, S. Woloshin, H. G. Welch.

> Drafting of the article：L. M. Schwartz, S. Woloshin.

> Critical revision of the article for important intellectual content：L. M. Schwartz, S. Woloshin, H. G. Welch.

> Obtaining of funding：S. Woloshin.

> Administrative, technical, or logistic support：S. Woloshin.

> Final approval of the article：L. M. Schwartz, S. Woloshin, H. G. Welch.

> Statistical expertise：L. M. Schwartz, S. Woloshin.

利益冲突说明（Conflict-of-interest disclosure）：要重视利益冲突说明。故意不披露利益冲突是一种科研不端行为。

公众对科学研究过程的信任和已发表论文的可信度，部分取决于在进行科学研究的作者和研究中使用到的药品、仪器、器械、资金的提供者是否有利益关联以及利益关联是否得到充分披露。利益关联并不代表一定会影响研究的可信度，但一定要公开，使读者有机会独立判断作者的利益关联是否会影响研究的可信度。

经济关系是最容易确认、最常见的利益冲突，包括雇佣关系、收取顾问费、购买了相关公司的股权或期权、专利交易以及有偿的专家代言。

如果没有可以陈述为：

> The authors declare no competing financial interests.

第6节　平行对照随机临床试验报告指南（CONSORT 声明）

随机对照临床试验是评价医疗干预措施效果的金标准。临床试验报告不充分会误导读者。1996 年"临床试验报告的统一标准（Consolidated Standards of Reporting Trials，CONSORT）声明"（简称 CONSORT 声明）的出台就是为了促进临床研究的可读性和可靠性。该声明的应用提高了随机对照临床试验的报告质量[2]。

"CONSORT 声明"包括有 25 项条目的论文撰写内容清单和一张流程图。"CONSORT 声明"针对最常用的两组平行随机对照试验，其他试验类型可以参考。CONSORT 相关文件可以从 CONSORT 网站（http://www.consortstatement.org）获取。

CONSORT 一直以来都获得众多出版社和机构的支持。ICMJE 和世界医学编辑协会（World Association of Medical Editors）均支持 CONSORT。因此，在向相关的期刊投稿的时候必须遵循 CONSORT 的撰写要求（表1.2）。

表 1.2　CONSORT 2010 对照检查清单

论文章节/主题	条目号	对照检查的条目
	1a	文题能识别是随机临床试验
	1b	结构式摘要，包括试验设计、方法、结果、结论几个部分
背景和目的	2a	科学背景和对试验理由的解释
	2b	具体目的和假设
试验设计	3a	描述试验设计（诸如平行设计、析因设计），包括受试者分配入各组的比例
	3b	试验开始后对试验方法所作的重要改变（如合格受试者的挑选标准），并说明原因
受试者	4a	受试者合格标准
	4b	资料收集的场所和地点
干预措施	5	详细描述各组干预措施的细节以使他人能够重复，包括它们实际上是在何时、如何实施的

论文章节/主题	条目号	对照检查的条目
结局指标	6a	完整而确切地说明预先设定的主要和次要结局指标,包括它们是在何时、如何测评的
	6b	试验开始后对结局指标是否有任何更改,并说明原因
样本量	7a	如何确定样本量
	7b	必要时,解释中期分析和试验中止原则

随机方法:

论文章节/主题	条目号	对照检查的条目
序列的产生	8a	产生随机分配序列的方法
	8b	随机方法的类型,任何限定的细节(如怎样分区组和各区组样本多少)
分配隐藏机制	9	用于执行随机分配序列的机制(例如按序编码的封藏法),描述干预措施分配之前为隐藏序列号所采取的步骤
实施	10	谁产生随机分配序列,谁招募受试者,谁给受试者分配干预措施
盲法	11a	如果实施了盲法,分配干预措施之后对谁设盲(例如受试者、医护提供者、结局评估者),以及盲法是如何实施的
	11b	如有必要,描述干预措施的相似之处
统计学方法	12a	用于比较各组主要和次要结局指标的统计学方法
	12b	附加分析的方法,诸如亚组分析和校正分析
受试者流程(极力推荐使用流程图)	13a	随机分配到各组的受试者例数,接受已分配治疗的例数,以及纳入主要结局分析的例数
	13b	随机分组后,各组脱落和被剔除的例数,并说明原因
招募受试者	14a	招募期和随访时间的长短,并说明具体日期
	14b	为什么试验中断或停止
基线资料	15	用一张表格列出每一组受试者的基线数据,包括人口学资料和临床特征
纳入分析的例数	16	各组纳入每一种分析的受试者数目(分母),以及是否按最初的分组分析
结局和估计值	17a	各组每一项主要和次要结局指标的结果,效应估计值及其精确性(如 95% 可信区间)
	17b	对于二分类结局,建议同时提供相对效应值和绝对效应值

论文章节/主题	条目号	对照检查的条目
辅助分析	18	所做的其他分析的结果,包括亚组分析和校正分析,指出哪些是预先设定的分析,哪些是新尝试的分析
危害	19	各组出现的所有严重危害或意外效果(具体的指导建议参见"CONSORT for harms")
局限性	20	试验的局限性,报告潜在偏倚和不精确的原因,以及出现多种分析结果的原因(如果有这种情况的话)
可推广性	21	试验结果被推广的可能性(外部可靠性,实用性)
解释	22	与结果相对应的解释,权衡试验结果的利弊,并且考虑其他相关证据
其他信息		
试验注册	23	临床试验注册号和注册机构名称
试验方案	24	如果有的话,在哪里可以获取完整的试验方案
资助	25	资助和其他支持(如提供药品)的来源,提供资助者所起的作用

CONSORT 不是对论文的格式进行标准化。文章的格式应该遵从期刊的风格、所涉及的研究领域的传统习惯,或作者的偏好。CONSORT 只要求作者在文中包括清单条目中的项目,并且足够详细地描述,强调报告要完整、清晰和透明化,即要反映试验设计、实施和结果的真实情况。

第 7 节　排版细则

页码

有些杂志要求从标题页开始标页码,有些杂志则从正文(text)开始标页码。页码的位置包括左、中和右,作者必须遵照杂志的要求。有些杂志还要求每行编码,以方便审稿的时候审稿人标注需要评论的内容所在的位置。

行距

一般来说,论文的行距(Line space)都是双倍行距(double-spaced),包括摘要、图标题以及参考文献。不要在段落之前或之后添加额外的行距。

但为了获得最好、最有效的布局,表格(单元格)可以是单倍行距、1.5 倍行距或双倍行距;图形、图像中的文字也可以是单倍行距、1.5 倍行距或双倍行距。

注意:"double-space"是动词,形容词用"double-spaced":

➢ In general, we double-space all parts of a paper。

≫ 段落对齐

对于段落对齐(paragraph alignment)的方式,一般是左对齐(Flush left),右边距不要对齐(Uneven or ragged)。不要使用两边对齐方式(Full justification)。不要在行尾插入连字符和手动换行符(Manual breaks)。但是文字处理程序自动在长超链接(例如参考文献的 DOI 或 URL)中插入中断是可以的。

≫ 段落缩进

每种杂志的段落缩进(Paragraph indentation)方式有差异。一般每段文字的第一行要缩进。但英式论文的第一段不缩进。

段落缩进一定要使用制表键(Tab key)或文字处理程序的自动段落格式化功能来实现缩进。不要使用空格键(Space bar)手动创建缩进。

有些例外情况,如:

标题页:标题、署名和单位名称不缩进,或者居中。

节标签(Section labels,如 Abstract、References):不缩进,或者居中。

摘要:摘要的第一行一般不缩进。

整段引用(Block quotation):从左边距缩进整段。如果有多个被引用的段落,则第二个段落开始的每个段落的第一行也要缩进。

表格和图表的标题和注释:左对齐,不缩进。

一般图和表格在投稿的时候单独上传。有时为了审稿方便,杂志会要求在文章没有接受前把图和表格放在文章中第一次提到的位置(Called out),在文章正式接受后再单独提交图和表。

≫ 注释

有的杂志要求注释(Footnotes)放在相应页的底部,有的杂志要求统一放在参考文献后面。

第8节 段落结构

段落是文章的基本组成部分。段落不是简单的句子堆积。结构良好的段落不仅有一个主题,而且会围绕这个主题展开。科技论文的段落在文章不同部分其长度显著不同。前言和讨论部分一般四到五句话。通常第一句话会介绍主题。其他句子可能给出定义、示例、原因和总结。每句话不要超过30个单词。方法和结果的段落则可长可短,根据内容来定,原则是一个段落包含相似的内容。

在前言和讨论部分,为了清楚起见,每个段落只讨论一个主题。段落的主题在段落的第一句出现。这个句子也叫主题句(Topic sentence)。确保每个句子都与主题句相关。如下面这个段落由 4 部分组成(Topic sentence,Example 1,Example 2 和 Summary):

段落结构	内容
1. Topic sentence	In 2000, using a glucocorticoid-free immunosuppressive protocol that included sirolimus, low-dose tacrolimus, and a monoclonal antibody against the interleukin-2 receptor (IL-2R) (daclizumab), Shapiro et al. carried out islet transplantation alone for seven patients with type 1 diabetes and a history of severe hypoglycemia and metabolic instability.
2. Example 1	They demonstrated that islet transplantation can result in insulin independence with excellent metabolic control when glucocorticoid-free immunosuppression is combined with the infusion of an adequate islet mass. This treatment became known as the Edmonton Protocol.
3. Example 2	As of 1 November 2004, 65 patients have received islet transplants at the University of Alberta, and results have been promising: the majority(80%) of the recipients have had C-peptide present following islet transplant.
4. Summary	Unfortunately, the median duration of insulin independence has been 15 months, and only a minority (10%) have maintained insulin independence 5 years following islet transplant.

段落之间要采用一些词联系起来，如：

Despite this…

XXX is another area for consideration…

Finally，the performance of…

第9节　词、词组和句子的并列

词和词组的并列用逗号分开，最后的词和词组前加 and 或者 or，如：

➤ The response of Fanca bone marrow to *in vitro* stimulation is characterized by (a) an accelerated depletion in CFU-GM progenitors，(b) an evident granulocyte/macrophage differentiation disbalance，and (c) a marked susceptibility of the expanded population to enter into apoptosis.

并列的句子则用句号分开，数字加括号，如：

➤ (1) IVIG(black IgGs) and 7E3(white IgGs) are taken into the cell by pinocytosis. (2) At physiologic pH，IgG has low affinity for the FcRn receptor. (3) Bound IgG molecules are protected from release into the lysosome.

或者用段落的格式，数字不加括号，后面加句号和空格。如：

1. IVIG(black IgGs) and 7E3(white IgGs) are taken into the cell by pinocytosis.

2. At physiologic pH，IgG has low affinity for the FcRn receptor.

3. Bound IgG molecules are protected from release into the lysosome.

参考文献

[1] Audisio R A，Stahel R A，Aapro M S，et al. Successful publishing：how to get your paper accepted[J]. Surg Oncol，2009，18：350 – 56.

[2] ICMJE Recommendations for the Conduct，Reporting，Editing，and Publication of Scholarly Work in Medical Journals[EB/OL]. https：//www. icmje. org/icmje – recommendations. pdf.

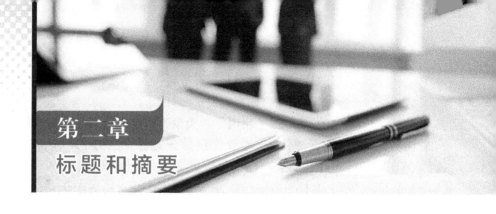

第1节 标 题

什么是好的标题？不同的人从不同的角度出发会有不同的观点。

在广告行业，人们常说广告必须在不到一秒的时间内吸引读者的注意力。好的论文标题也是如此。当然论文的标题不能像广告那样通过花哨、夸张的语言吸引读者，读者毕竟不是普通消费者。对于一篇内容精彩的论文，标题如果能够充分描述论文的内容，并让读者想阅读论文，那么它就是好的。

一位资深编辑这样说：好的标题是杂志编辑认为好的标题。这句话很有道理。对标题的评估在很大程度上是一个主观问题，不同的期刊有不同的规则和做法。许多期刊，如《NEJM》，不接受声明性标题，即揭示研究结果或结论的标题。这种做法似乎越来越得到认可。

有人认为一个好标题是用尽可能少的单词充分描述文章内容的标题（包括结果）。短标题通常比长标题更可取。《BMJ》的编辑曾列出她对一个好标题的要求：简洁、准确、具体、不误导和不遗漏重要信息（例如要包含研究类型）。

不管如何，以下规则是普遍适用的：

（1）题目足够精确以便他人能够在数据库中检索到。

（2）标题中不要挤进太多信息和太多长词。如果初稿标题太长，最好先列出标题中的单词优先顺序，然后再优化，做到只包含（或几乎只包含）优先级最高的单词，如：The effects of SU11248 on human tumor xenografts: an *in vivo* study，可以改为：Oral sunitinib inhibits growth of human tumor xenografts。

（3）除非有副标题，否则不使用标点符号。不使用缩写。如果标题中包含了通俗易懂的缩写，也必须在摘要中对其进行定义。

（4）如果文章只报道了使用非人类模型的研究结果，那么必须在标题中注明物种，以免误导读者（笔者曾经碰到这样的标题：A novel method of tracheal anastomosis healing using a single submucosal injection of basic fibroblast growth factor：initial report。看上去像是临床研究，因此很感兴趣，但看了才知道是动物研究，令人失望）。

（5）标题最好是短语，但如有必要，可以是陈述句或疑问句，这时候一般用主动语态。

（6）如果标题中提到药物名称，则应使用通用名称（Generic name），除非文章是针对不同公司的同一药品进行比较，或文章对特定公司的药物进行研究和评论。

（7）随机对照研究（Randomized controlled trial，RCT）的标题一般要把对照组写出来，如：

➢ Effect of high-flow nasal cannula therapy vs continuous positive airway pressure following extubation on liberation from respiratory support in critically ill children：a randomized clinical trial。

但如果对照组是显然易见的时候，也可以不写，如：

➢ Effect of alirocumab added to high-intensity stain therapy on coronary atherosclerosis in patients with acute myocardial infarction：the PACMAN-AMI randomized clinical trial。

这里作者注明了研究组是"high-intensity statin therapy"基础上增加"（add on）alirocumab"，因此对照组是"high-intensity statin therapy"。作者强调了新的治疗方案。

再如：

➢ Effect of sotrovimab on hospitalization or death among high-risk patients with mild to moderate COVID-19：a randomized clinical trial

➢ Effect of antiplatelet therapy on survival and organ support-free days in critically ill patients with COVID-19：a randomized clinical trial

临床研究的标题通常含以下内容："Effect of（干预方法）on（in，for）（疗效指标）among（in）patients with（疾病）：（研究类型）"，如上面的两个例子（Effect of sotrovimab on hospitalization…；Effect of antiplatelet therapy on survival…）。

另外一种常见的标题的格式特点是："Safety and efficacy of（干预方法）

on(in，for)（疗效指标）among（in）patients with(疾病)：(研究类型)"。如：

> Safety and efficacy of prednisone versus placebo in short-term prevention of episodic cluster headache：a multicentre，double-blind，randomised controlled trial

> Safety and efficacy of amantadine，modafinil，and methylphenidate for fatigue in multiple sclerosis：a randomised，placebo-controlled，crossover，double-blind trial

> Safety and efficacy of amantadine，modafinil，and methylphenidate for fatigue in multiple sclerosis：a randomised，placebo-controlled，crossover，double-blind trial

> Long-term safety and efficacy of patisiran for hereditary transthyretin-mediated amyloidosis with polyneuropathy：12-month results of an open-label extension study

《NEJM》沿用简洁的标题,其特点是只包含干预方法和疾病。对于随机对照研究,这样的标题是不符合"CONSORT 声明"的,但"老大"就是任性。如：

> Rilzabrutinib，an Oral BTK Inhibitor，in Immune Thrombocytopenia

> Neoadjuvant Nivolumab plus Chemotherapy in Resectable Lung Cancer

> Ivosidenib and Azacitidine in IDH1-Mutated Acute Myeloid Leukemia

> Mitapivat versus Placebo for Pyruvate Kinase Deficiency

初写论文的作者会不自觉采用以下句式,应避免：

> A study of…

> A report of a case of…

> An investigation into…

这些句式一般用于毕业论文的标题。

第 2 节　摘　要

审稿人对论文的最初了解来自摘要。杂志社邀请审稿人的时候也是先通过电子邮件发稿件的摘要给审稿人,以便审稿人根据研究内容决定是否接受邀请。摘要写得不好,或者文字和语法错误太多,或者审稿人无法读懂而导致拒绝审稿邀请,导致审稿延迟;也可能在编辑部初审的时候遭到直接拒稿。

摘要一般 250～300 字,并以逻辑顺序简洁地陈述研究的基本原理(或假设、目标)、方法、结果和结论。

摘要不包含参考文献,尽可能避免使用行话和缩略词,确保读者容易阅读和理解。

根据 ICMJE 建议,研究论文的摘要包含以下内容:

- 研究的背景或目的。清楚地描述背景和目的,即为什么进行该研究。(1～2 句)

- 方法包括研究参与者的选择、医院类型、疗效指标、分析方法。(3～4 句)

- 主要发现,给出具体的效应大小。(3～5 句)

- 主要结论和对研究结果的解释,强调研究的重要性。(2～3 句)

下面我们以在《NEJM》发表的一篇题目为"A randomized trial of tai chi for fibromyalgia"的论文为例说明这些要素[1]。文章报告了一项采用太极拳治疗纤维肌痛的随机对照研究。第一作者为美国塔夫茨大学医学院医学中心风湿病科的 Chenchen Wang 博士。

摘要一共有 4 个部分。第一部分如下:

Background:*Previous research has suggested that tai chi offers a therapeutic benefit in patients with fibromyalgia.*

背景 先前的研究表明,太极拳对纤维肌痛患者有治疗作用。

该部分只有一句,采用现在完成时,提示太极拳以前用于纤维肌痛,现在还在用,也提示本研究将涉及太极拳和纤维肌痛。

Methods *We conducted a single-blind, randomized trial of classic Yang-style tai chi as compared with a control intervention consisting of wellness education and stretching for the treatment of fibromyalgia (defined by American College of Rheumatology 1990 criteria). Sessions lasted 60 minutes each and took place twice a week for 12 weeks for each of the study groups. The primary end point was a change in the Fibromyalgia Impact Questionnaire(FIQ) score(ranging from 0 to 100, with higher scores indicating more severe symptoms) at the end of 12 weeks. Secondary end points included summary scores on the physical and mental components of the Medical Outcomes Study 36-Item Short-Form Health Survey(SF-36). All assessments were repeated at 24 weeks to test the durability of the response.*

方法 我们对经典杨式太极拳进行了一项单盲随机试验,并与健康教育和拉伸活动进行了治疗纤维肌痛(按照美国风湿病学会 1990 年标准诊断)的对照研究。每个研究组每次持续 60 分钟,每周进行两次,为期 12 周。主要终点是 12 周结束时纤维肌痛影响问卷(FIQ)评分的变化(从 0 到 100,评分越高表示症状越严重)。次要终点包括 36 项简短健康调查(SF-36)的身体和心理部分的汇总分数。在 24 周时重复所有评估,以测试疗效的持久性。

方法描述了研究参与者的分组、干预方法、观察时间点、主要和次要疗效指标。用过去时。

Results *Of the 66 randomly assigned patients, the 33 in the tai chi group had clinically important improvements in the FIQ total score and quality of life. Mean($\pm$SD) baseline and 12-week FIQ scores for the tai chi group were 62.9 $\pm$15.5 and 35.1 $\pm$18.8, respectively, versus 68.0 $\pm$11 and 58.6 $\pm$17.6, respectively, for the control group(change from baseline in the tai chi group vs. change from baseline in the control group, -18.4 points; $P < 0.001$). The corresponding SF-36 physical-component scores were 28.5 $\pm$8.4 and 37.0 $\pm$10.5 for the tai chi group versus 28.0 $\pm$7.8 and 29.4 $\pm$7.4 for the control group(between-group difference, 7.1 points; $P = 0.001$), and the mental-component scores were 42.6 $\pm$12.2 and 50.3 $\pm$10.2 for the tai chi group versus 37.8 $\pm$10.5 and 39.4 $\pm$11.9 for the control group (between-group difference, 6.1 points; $P = 0.03$). Improvements were maintained at 24 weeks(between-group difference in the FIQ score, -18.3 points; $P < 0.001$). No adverse events were observed.*

结果 在 66 名随机分配的患者中,太极拳组的 33 名患者在 FIQ 总分和生活质量方面有临床上重要的改善。太极组的基线和 12 周平均($\pm$SD)FIQ 评分分别为 62.9$\pm$15.5 和 35.1$\pm$18.8,而对照组为 68.0$\pm$11 和 58.6$\pm$17.6(太极组的基线变化与对照组的基线变化的差异,-18.4 分;$P < 0.001$)。太极组的基线和 12 周 SF-36 身体成分得分分别为 28.5$\pm$8.4 和 37.0$\pm$10.5,而对照组为 28.0$\pm$7.8 和 29.4$\pm$7.4(组间差异,7.1 分;$P = 0.001$),太极组的心理成分得分分别为 42.6$\pm$12.2 和 50.3$\pm$10.2,而对照组为 37.8$\pm$10.5 和 39.4$\pm$11.9(组间差异,6.1 分;$P = 0.03$)。24 周时仍有改善(FIQ 得分组间差异为 -18.3 分;$P < 0.001$)。未观察到不良事件。

结果包括入组患者人数,依次描述主要疗效、次要疗效和不良反应。描述疗效的时候先描述研究组,再描述对照组。用过去时。

Conclusions *Tai chi may be a useful treatment for fibromyalgia and merits long-term study in larger study populations. (Funded by the National Center for Complementary and Alternative Medicine and others;*

ClinicalTrials. gov number，NCT00515008）

结论　太极拳可能是治疗纤维肌痛的有效方法，值得在更大的研究人群中进行长期研究（由国家补充和替代医学中心等资助；ClinicalTrials. gov 注册号：NCT00515008）。

这里作者强调结论的普适性，采用现在时。临床试验注册信息一般在摘要的最后一句给出。

下面我们再举一个例子[2]：

Background　*Pyruvate kinase deficiency is a rare，hereditary，chronic condition that is associated with hemolytic anemia. In a phase 2 study，mitapivat，an oral，first-in-class activator of erythrocyte pyruvate kinase，increased the hemoglobin level in patients with pyruvate kinase deficiency.*

背景　丙酮酸激酶缺乏症是一种罕见的遗传性慢性疾病，与溶血性贫血有关。在一项 2 期研究中，mitapivat，一种口服的、同类首个红细胞丙酮酸激酶激活剂，增加了丙酮酸激酶缺乏症患者的血红蛋白水平。

第一句是常识，因此用现在时。第二句用过去式介绍已经完成了 2 期研究的内容，既是背景介绍，也提示本研究将是 3 期临床研究。

"First in Class"指按照某个药理学机制研发的、治疗某种疾病的第一个新药。

Methods　*In this global，phase 3，randomized，placebo-controlled trial，we evaluated the efficacy and safety of mitapivat in adults with pyruvate kinase deficiency who were not receiving regular red-cell transfusions. The patients were assigned to receive either mitapivat（5 mg twice daily，with potential escalation to 20 or 50 mg twice daily）or placebo for 24 weeks. The primary end point was a hemoglobin response（an increase from baseline of ≥1.5 g per deciliter in the hemoglobin level）that was sustained at two or more scheduled assessments at weeks 16，20，and 24. Secondary efficacy end points were the average change from baseline in the hemoglobin level，markers of hemolysis and hematopoiesis，and the change from baseline at week 24 in two pyruvate kinase deficiency-specific patient-reported outcome measures.*

方法　在这项全球 3 期随机安慰剂对照试验中，我们评估了 mitapivat 在未接受常规红细胞输注的丙酮酸激酶缺乏症成人中的疗效和安全性。患者被分配接受 mitapivat（每天两次，每次 5 mg，可增加到每天两次，每次 20 mg

或 50 mg)或安慰剂治疗 24 周。主要终点是在第 16、20 和 24 周的两次或两次以上计划评估中持续的血红蛋白增加(血红蛋白水平比基线增加≥1.5 g/dL)。次要疗效终点是血红蛋白水平、溶血和造血标志物与基线的平均变化,以及第 24 周丙酮酸激酶缺乏症患者报告的两种结果指标与基线的变化。)

方法包括研究参与者的分组、用药方法、观察时间点、主要和次要疗效指标。用过去时。

Results Sixteen of the 40 patients(40%) in the mitapivat group had a hemoglobin response, as compared with none of the 40 patients in the placebo group (adjusted difference, 39.3 percentage points; 95% confidence interval, 24.1 to 54.6; two-sided $P < 0.001$). Patients who received mitapivat had a greater response than those who received placebo with respect to each secondary end point, including the average change from baseline in the hemoglobin level. The most common adverse events were nausea(in 7 patients [18%] in the mitapivat group and 9 patients [23%] in the placebo group) and headache(in 6 patients [15%] and 13 patients [33%], respectively). Adverse events of grade 3 or higher occurred in 10 patients(25%) who received mitapivat and 5 patients(13%) who received placebo.

结果 Mitapivat 组 40 名患者中有 16 名(40%)有血红蛋白增加,而安慰剂组 40 名病人中没有(调整后差异,39.3 个百分点;95%置信区间,24.1 至 54.6;双侧 $P < 0.001$)。次要指标方面,全部指标 mitapivat 组都优于安慰剂组,包括血红蛋白水平与基线的平均变化。最常见的不良事件是恶心[mitapivat 组 7 名患者(18%),安慰剂组 9 名患者(23%)]和头痛[分别为 6 名患者(15%)和 13 名患者(33%)]。10 名(25%)接受 mitapivat 治疗的患者和 5 名(13%)接受安慰剂治疗的患者发生了 3 级或更高的不良事件。

结果包括入组患者人数,依次描述主要疗效、次要疗效和不良反应。描述疗效的时候百分数和病例数都要注明,如"in 6 patients [15%] and 13 patients [33%], respectively"。应用过去时。

Conclusions In patients with pyruvate kinase deficiency, mitapivat significantly increased the hemoglobin level, decreased hemolysis, and improved patient-reported outcomes. No new safety signals were identified in the patients who received mitapivat. (Funded by Agios Pharmaceuticals; ClinicalTrials. gov number, NCT03548220.)

结论 在丙酮酸激酶缺乏症患者中,mitapivat 显著提高了血红蛋白水平,减少了溶血,改善了患者报告的结果。在接受 mitapivat 治疗的患者中没有发现新的不良反应(由 Agios 制药公司资助;ClinicalTrials.gov 注册号:NCT03548220)。

和上一个摘要不同,这里主要结论用过去时,目的是强调此次研究的结果。

有些老牌杂志还沿用一段式摘要,或者其他格式的摘要,但要求的内容都是一样的。如《Lancet》的摘要包括以下部分:Background、Methods、Findings(对应 Results)和 Interpretation(对应 Conclusion)。

《Nature》的格式采用一段式,而且允许用参考文献。尤其是它允许整个摘要采用现在时描述研究的结果,不带具体数字,因为作者认为这些结果很肯定,如[3]:

SARS-CoV-2 is a single-stranded RNA virus that causes COVID-19. Given its acute and often self-limiting course, it is likely that components of the innate immune system play a central part in controlling virus replication and determining clinical outcome. Natural killer (NK) cells are innate lymphocytes with notable activity against a broad range of viruses, including RNA viruses[1,2]. NK cell function may be altered during COVID-19 despite increased representation of NK cells with an activated and adaptive phenotype[3,4]. Here we show that a decline in viral load in COVID-19 correlates with NK cell status and that NK cells can control SARS-CoV-2 replication by recognizing infected target cells. In severe COVID-19, NK cells show defects in virus control, cytokine production and cell-mediated cytotoxicity despite high expression of cytotoxic effector molecules. Single-cell RNA sequencing of NK cells over the time course of the COVID-19 disease spectrum reveals a distinct gene expression signature. Transcriptional networks of interferon-driven NK cell activation are superimposed by a dominant transforming growth factor-β (TGFβ) response signature, with reduced expression of genes related to cell-cell adhesion, granule exocytosis and cell-mediated cytotoxicity. In severe COVID-19, serum levels of TGFβ peak during the first two weeks of infection, and serum obtained from these patients severely inhibits NK cell function in a TGFβ-dependent manner. Our data reveal that an untimely production of TGFβ is a hallmark of severe COVID-19 and may inhibit NK cell function and early control of the virus.

SARS-CoV-2 是一种引起新冠感染的单链 RNA 病毒。鉴于其急性且经常自限性的过程,先天免疫系统的组成部分很可能在控制病毒复制和决定临床转归方面发挥着核心作用。自然杀伤(NK)细胞是天然的淋巴细胞,对多种病毒(包括 RNA 病毒[1,2])具有显著活性。尽管具有活化和适应性表型的 NK 细胞的比例增加,但在新冠感染期间 NK 细胞功能可能会发生改变[3,4]。在这里,我们表明,新冠病毒载量的下降与 NK 细胞状态相关,NK 细胞可以通过识别受感染的靶细胞来控制 SARS-CoV-2 的复制。在严重的新冠肺炎感染中,尽管细胞毒效应分子高表达,但 NK 细胞在病毒控制、细胞因子产生和细胞介导的细胞毒性方面仍存在缺陷。在新冠感染进程中,NK 细胞的单细胞 RNA 测序揭示了一个独特的基因表达特征。干扰素驱动的 NK 细胞激活的转录网络与显性转化生长因子-β(TGF-β)反应信号叠加,与细胞间黏附、颗粒胞吐和细胞介导的细胞毒性相关的基因表达减少。在严重的新冠感染患者中,TGF-β 的血清水平在前两个周达到峰值。这些患者的血清以 TGFβ 依赖的方式明显抑制 NK 细胞功能。我们的数据表明,TGFβ 的过早生成是严重新冠肺炎的标志,可能会抑制 NK 细胞功能和病毒的早期控制。

　　所以对摘要的格式,一定要"入乡随俗",尤其是准备在老牌杂志上发表的论文。

　　有些杂志要求写要点(Key points),一般 3～5 条,每条 1 行。要点放在摘要的前面,不编入 PubMed 等数据库。要点概括研究的最重要结果、意义及其对读者的价值。要点尽量不要用晦涩的专业词汇。

　　最后,越来越多的期刊要求作者提供图文摘要(Graphic abstract)。图文摘要大致分为 2 种形式。一种是用一张图描述论文的核心内容,如图 2.1:

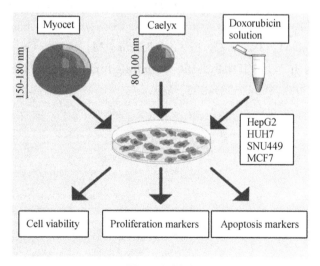

图 2.1　例图

还有一种是包含摘要的主要内容，如图 2.2：

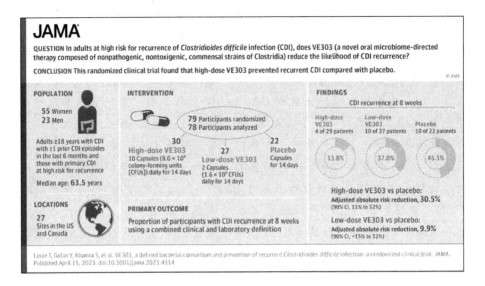

图 2.2　例图

参考文献

［1］ Wang C，Schmid C H，Rones R，et al. A randomized trial of tai chi for fibromyalgia［J］. N Engl J Med. 2010，363(8)：743 - 754.

［2］ Al-Samkari H，Galactéros F，Glenthøj A，et al. Mitapivat versus Placebo for Pyruvate Kinase Deficiency［J］. N Engl J Med. 2022，386 (15)：1432 - 1442.

［3］ Witkowski M，Tizian C，Ferreira-Gomes M，et al. Untimely TGFβ responses in COVID-19 limit antiviral functions of NK cells［J］. Nature. 2021，600(7888)：295 - 301.

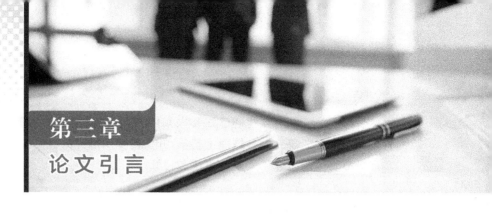

引言也就是开场白,目的是向读者提供所研究的课题的基本信息,包括课题相关的基本知识(背景)、研究的目的(研究针对的具体问题)和方法。它通过总结到目前为止的相关文献向审稿人和读者介绍研究的背景。对于作者本人的系列研究,要重点介绍本人的前期研究结果。一个好的引言,内容上要体现课题的创新性,抓住编辑、审稿人和读者的眼球,同时语言描述上具有逻辑性,让阅读者读起来很轻松,所谓的"Be nice to reviewers"。

引言可以在研究开始时,甚至研究开始前就撰写。

第 1 节　引言的结构

我们要清楚,审稿人虽然是相关领域的专家,但对作者研究的具体问题不一定非常熟悉。比如,同样是肿瘤学专家,你研究的信号通路审稿专家可能不熟悉。因此引言必须让审稿人了解本研究的生物学、临床或方法学原理。通过清晰的介绍获得审稿人对研究的认可是论文获得好评的第一步。

引言主要包含的内容是:

1. 研究背景和问题陈述。

2. 研究问题、研究目的或假设。

3. 所采取方法的概述。

引言的结构可以看成一个漏斗。顶部是最宽泛的部分(开头),描写研究的大背景,如研究的疾病的定义,目前的治疗方法,强调疾病对个人健康、家庭经济和社会负担的严重影响,目前的治疗方法的不足之处等。背景介绍的段落通常以结论或问题的陈述结束,为即将研究的特定问题设置一个伏笔。例如:

➢ The disease is poorly understood.

➢ New treatment is needed.

然后概述关于特定主题的已知和未知的知识,将范围缩小到更具主题性的背景和本论文的研究的具体理论基础,并由此提出研究的目标或假说。

最后简要提出研究将采用的方法和目标。

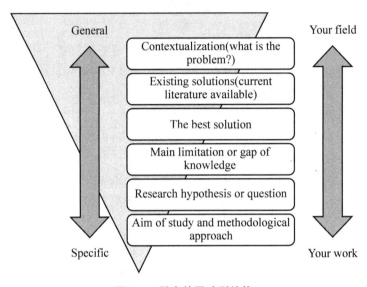

图 3.1　引言的漏斗型结构

因此,引言可以按照以下段落布局:

第一段是大背景(General)。其中第一句应该包含论文标题中的大部分单词,阐明论文所涉及的问题,以满足读者的期望并保持他们的注意力。

第二段应为本研究提供更具体(Specific)的背景和动机。通常做一个临床研究有两个原因:

(1) 研究(或试验)是一系列研究中合乎逻辑的下一步,如:从 1 期临床研究到 2 期临床研究,从 2 期临床研究到 3 期临床研究。

(2) 先前的研究在某种程度上存在无法避免的缺陷或局限性,而当前的研究目标是解决这一问题,如从回顾性研究到前瞻性研究、从概念验证研究(Proof of concept,PoC)研究到 RCT、从小样本研究到大样本研究、从单中心研究到多中心研究、从 A 种族到 B 种族研究、从单一疾病人群研究到多疾病人群研究(如研究某种降糖药对糖尿病合并高血压人群的降糖效果)、从单一药物治疗到复方或多种药物治疗(理论上疗效更好)的研究、采用新的疗效指标的研究、从成年人到儿童(或老人、孕妇)和短期疗效到延长随访时间的长期疗效的研究,等等。

如果是第一个原因,那么背景文献应该关注最重要的 2~4 篇相关研究的文章,并合乎逻辑地展示是如何导致你目前的研究的。如果是第二个原因,则应引用 2~4 项最重要的、有"缺陷"的研究,并明确说明其不足之处和你的目的。

通常在引用参考文献的时候避免提及作者(例如:Anderson et al reported that…)以增强文字的流畅,避免累赘。

第三段应该明确说明需要进行研究的主要目的、期望解决的问题或假设。不要担心公式化、模式化的写作,科技论文都是这样。忙碌的审稿人希望开门见山。

第四段简单介绍将采用的方法和预期结果。

第三或第四段一般要包含类似"The purpose of this study was to…"的句子。

下面我们以"A randomized trial of tai chi for fibromyalgia"为例介绍引言如何展开[1]。文章报告了一项采用太极拳治疗纤维肌痛的 RCT。

The NEW ENGLAND JOURNAL of MEDICINE

ORIGINAL ARTICLE

A Randomized Trial of Tai Chi for Fibromyalgia

文章的前言一共有 4 段。第一段如下:

Fibromyalgia is a common and complex clinical syndrome characterized by chronic and widespread musculoskeletal pain, fatigue, sleep disturbance, and physical and psychological impairment.[1,2] Evidence-based guidelines suggest that fibromyalgia is typically managed with multidisciplinary therapies involving medication, cognitive behavioral therapy, education, and exercise.[3-5]

纤维肌痛是一种常见而复杂的综合征,其特征是慢性和广泛的肌肉骨骼疼痛、疲劳、睡眠障碍以及身体和心理不适[1,2]。基于循证医学的指南建议采用药物、认知行为疗法、教育和锻炼等综合治疗纤维肌痛[3-5]。

此段文字对纤维肌痛的特征和目前治疗方法做了全方位的介绍,相当于漏斗的顶部,而且包含了论文的主题:纤维肌痛(疾病)、疼痛(症状之一)和治疗方法,表明研究目的不是疾病的病理学,也不是流行病学,是治疗方法。治疗的对象是有纤维肌痛的疼痛患者。

作者采用了五篇参考文献,整段用现在时表示大家公认的知识。注意,超过三个名词并列,最后的"and"前面要加逗号。

第二段如下:

Although exercise is beneficial for fibromyalgia and has been advocated as a core component of its treatment,[6-8] most patients continue to be in considerable pain years after the original diagnosis and require medication to control symptoms; they also remain aerobically unfit, with poor muscle strength and limited flexibility.[9] New approaches are needed to reduce musculoskeletal pain in patients with fibromyalgia and to improve their physical and emotional functioning and quality of life.

尽管运动对纤维肌痛有益,并被推荐为治疗的主要方法[6-8],但大多数患者在诊断后数年内仍处于相当痛苦的状态,需要药物控制症状;他们仍然不适合有氧运动,肌肉力量差,柔韧性有限[9]。需要新的方法来减轻纤维肌痛患者的肌肉骨骼疼痛,改善他们的身体和精神以及生活质量。

第二段处于漏斗的中间,将话题收窄到运动治疗,通过四篇文献阐明现有运动治疗的不足,提示本研究将涉及新的运动治疗方法。注意,段落的第一句和最后一句有承上启下的作用。

这里作者用现在时表示大家公认的结论。此外"has been advocated"用的是现在完成时,表示过去开始但尚未完成,或还在进行,或未来很可能再次发生的行动,提示和现在有关联。

下面两句话也可以看出过去时和现在完成时的区别:

➢ The patient has been admitted to hospital two times(提示今天又来了).

➢ The patient was admitted to hospital two times(只描述过去的事实).

第三段如下:

Tai chi is a mind-body practice that originated in China as a martial art. It combines meditation with slow, gentle, graceful movements, as well as deep breathing and relaxation, to move vital energy (or qi) throughout the body. It is considered a complex, multicomponent intervention that integrates physical, psychosocial, emotional, spiritual, and behavioral elements.[10] Because of its mind-body attributes, tai chi could be especially well suited to the treatment of fibromyalgia. In fact, tai chi is practiced preferentially in the United States by persons with musculoskeletal and mental health conditions.[11,12] A small, nonrandomized study showed that tai chi reduced symptoms and improved quality of life in patients with fibromyalgia , 13 and it has also been shown to have potential therapeutic benefits in patients with other chronic rheumatic conditions , such as rheumatoid arthritis and osteoarthritis. [14,15]

太极拳是一种身心运动,起源于中国武术。它将冥想与缓慢、温和、优美的动作以及深呼吸和放松相结合,以运行全身的生命能量(或气)。它是一种综合了身体、心理、情感、精神和行为因素的复杂、多成分干预手段[10]。由于太极拳的身心属性,它特别适合治疗纤维肌痛。确实在美国有肌肉骨骼和心理健康问题的人喜欢打太极拳[11,12]。一项小型的非随机研究表明,太极拳可以减轻纤维肌痛患者的症状并提高生活质量[13],而且它也被证明对患有其他慢性风湿性疾病(如类风湿性关节炎和骨关节炎)的患者有潜在的益处[14,15]。

第三段处于漏斗的中下部位,继续将话题收窄到太极拳这个具体的运动形式上。该段介绍了太极拳的原理和临床实践,作为本临床研究的科学原理。同时用"A small, nonrandomized study"提示了现有研究的不足之处。

注意,在介绍太极拳的常识时候用现在时,但介绍具体的研究(A small, nonrandomized study showed)时用过去式。这里"condition"不是条件,是疾病的意思,但范围比"disease"更加宽泛(如:A condition indicates your state of health. It is an abnormal state that feels different from your normal state of wellbeing. Often, you'll hear about someone's condition when they are hospitalized and noted as being in stable or critical condition. 又如:Over the past few decades, the incidence of inflammatory and autoimmune conditions in Westernised nations has risen sharply)[2]。

第四段如下:

We conducted a single-blind , randomized , controlled trial to compare the physical and psychological benefits of tai chi with those of a control intervention that consisted of wellness education and stretching. We hypothesized that at the end of the 12-week intervention period , patients in the tai chi group would have a greater reduction in musculoskeletal pain and greater improvements in sleep quality , physical and psychological function , and health-related quality-of-life scores than those in the control group.

我们进行了一项单盲、随机、对照试验,以比较太极拳与健康教育和伸展运动组成的对照干预的身体和心理益处。我们的假设是,在12周干预结束时,太极拳组患者的肌肉骨骼疼痛将比对照组患者减轻得更多,睡眠质量、身体和心理功能以及健康相关生活质量评分也将得到更大改善。

该段作为最后一段,简要指出了本研究的方法(分组、随访时间和研究终点）。注意，中文通常会说"本研究将……"而英文则用过去时，因为计划是过去制定的，研究已经完成。

再如《JAMA》发表的一篇文章[3]：

Induction therapy, routinely implemented in organ transplant procedures, consists of biologic agents to block early immune activation. For kidney transplants, lymphodepletion with antithymocyte globulin (ATG) or alemtuzumab has contributed to reducing acute rejection episodes and improving early graft function but remains associated with toxic effects, cytomegalovirus reactivation, and posttransplant lymphoproliferative disease.

实施器官移植通常需要先进行诱导治疗，包括采用生物制剂阻断早期免疫激活。对于肾脏移植，用抗胸腺细胞球蛋白（ATG）或阿仑单抗清除淋巴细胞有助于减少急性排斥反应和改善早期移植肾功能，但会伴发不良反应、巨细胞病毒再激活和移植后淋巴增生性疾病。

这段的主题是介绍诱导治疗（Induction therapy）；然后举例，肾移植的时候常用的诱导治疗方法（ATG，alemtuzumab）；最后得出结论，即目前方法有不足之处。

然后概述关于特定主题的已知和未知的知识，将范围缩小到更具主题性的背景和本论文的研究的具体理论基础：

Novel induction immunosuppressive protocols with increased efficacy and minimal adverse effects are desirable. Appealing are the immunoregulatory properties of bone marrow-derived mesenchymal stem cells (MSCs), which represent a nonhematopoietic cell population that can differentiate into mesenchymal tissues (ie, bone, cartilage, or fat). They inhibit T-cell proliferation, monocyte differentiation to dendritic cells, modulate B-cell functions, and suppress natural killer cytotoxic effects. Thus, MSCs offer new therapeutic opportunities to prevent transplant rejection. Le Blanc et al first reported the striking clinical response to haploidentical MSCs in a case of severe, treatment-resistant grade IV acute graft-vs-host disease. A multicenter phase 2 trial for steroid-resistant, severe acute graft-vs-host disease confirmed this observation, while showing no adverse effects after MSC infusion. Mesenchymal stem cells obtained from either HLA-identical siblings, haploidentical, or HLA-mismatched third-party donors were similarly effective.

希望有新的、高效低毒的诱导免疫抑制方案。骨髓源性间充质干细胞（MSCs）的免疫调节作用很有前景，它是一种可以分化为间充质组织（即骨、软骨或脂肪）的非造血细胞。它有抑制 T 细胞增殖、单核细胞向树突状细胞分化、调节 B 细胞的功能，并抑制自然杀伤细胞毒性作用。因此，MSCs 为防止移植排斥提供了新的治疗机会。Le Blanc 等人首次报道了在一例严重的、耐药的 Ⅳ 级急性移植物抗宿主病病例中，半相合 MSCs 的显著临床疗效。一项针对类固醇耐药、严重急性移植物抗宿主病的多中心 2 期试验证实了这一观察结果，MSC 输注后没有出现不良反应。从 HLA 相同同胞、半相合或 HLA 不匹配的第三方供体获得的间充质干细胞同样有效。

第二段的第一句是该段的主题句（Novel … protocols … are desirable）。接下来通过举例介绍 MSC 的功能和已有的临床应用知识。

最后提出研究的目标或假说：

Our study aimed at examining the effect of autologous MSC infusion as an alternative to anti-IL-2 receptor antibody for induction therapy in adults undergoing living-related donor kidney transplants.

我们的研究旨在研究自体 MSC 输注作为抗 IL-2 受体抗体的替代药物在接受活体亲属肾移植的成人中作为诱导治疗的效果。

引言的最后一段是审稿人和读者最关注的内容。在这个部分要提出计划验证的假设，简要说明为了回答提出的问题计划做的工作，这也具有承上启下的作用，为方法部分创建一个很好的桥梁。

写完引言后，问问自己，审稿人是否明白了你为什么要进行这项研究，明白你的目的、目标是什么。以下清单供参考：

- What is the study all about?

- What is known and what is unknown about this specific subject?

- Why this study was needed, and why is it important?

- What is the primary research question? What did we want to know?

- What is the study design? What did you do to answer the research question?

要毫不犹豫地强调论文的研究的必要性和重要性。当全部作者一致认为把问题写得非常清楚时才能去投稿。

第2节 引言中需要注意的地方

在写引言的时候,注意以下原则:

- 引言尽可能简洁,通常不超过杂志的一页纸,占全文的 10%～15%。

- 讨论部分也可能会涉及背景知识,可以和引言有部分重叠。

- 明确区分主要和次要的研究问题。如果有次要的研究目标,一定要使用单独的句子明确指出。

- 尽量使用主动语态,并考虑使用信令词,例如:"to determine whether" "to clarify this""to compare"。

- 一般只用现在时、过去式和现在完成时。已建立的事实使用现在时态,例如:

> Low back pain is a common reason to consult physical therapists.

用过去时描述没有获得公认的结果或个别研究,例如:

> Two treatment sessions a week proved more beneficial than one session per week in a cohort study.

> In 1999 it was demonstrated that…

现在完成时可以表达特殊的意境,如过去开始、正在进行的行动,暗示过去的行动对现在有影响(未来很可能再次发生),例如:

> Exercise is beneficial for fibromyalgia and has been advocated as a core component of its treatment.

> I've seen the movie six times! [probably will see it again]

> I saw the movie six times! [probably will not see it again]

现在完成时和"recent","recently""just"或"now"一起使用则可以强调最近完成的动作 。尽管这一行动发生在过去,但它是如此之近,以至于它直接与现在联系在一起,例如:

> Interestingly, a similar knock-in murine model of the Tnnt2 K210Δ mutation has just been reported by Du and colleagues.

> Recently, we have demonstrated that spinal injection of fractalkine causes p38 activation.

> studies have demonstrated that neuroinflammation and ischemia can elicit two different types of reactive astrocytes, termed A1s and A2s.

现在完成时还可以强调一段时间内发生的变化,例如:

➢ Hypertension has been a great economic burden in the past 30 years.

如果是否定句,现在完成时强调了一个过去没有完成,现在将被完成的动作,如:

➢ To our knowledge, this finding has not been reported before.

➢ However, its antidepressant-like effect has not been reported before (so far, previously).

➢ The disease has not been reported in adults.

在结论中使用现在完成时可以让过去的动作听起来更重要。

➢ Macbeth has killed the king.

➢ We have demonstrated that increasing the dose of aspirin would cause bleeding.

• 最后通常使用过去时态介绍假设和工作计划。

• 一般不描述研究结果。

• 通过引用文献支持重要的结论时,确保引用真正相关的原始文献。有些杂志希望引用自身期刊中的相关论文,一方面表示你是他们的杂志的读者,另外可以提高杂志的影响因子(前提是引用近两年的文章)。

参考文献

[1] Wang C, Schmid C H, Rones R, et al. A randomized trial of tai chi for fibromyalgia[J]. N Engl J Med, 2010,363(8):743-754.

[2] https://www. differencebetween. com/difference-between-condition-and-vs-disease/.

[3] Tan J, Wu W, Xu X, et al. Induction therapy with autologous mesenchymal stem cells in living-related kidney transplants: a randomized controlled trial [J]. JAMA, 2012,307(11):1169-1177.

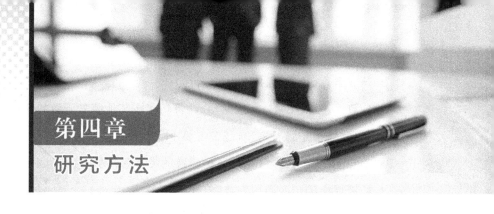

第四章
研究方法

　　如果把研究结果比喻为菜肴,那么一篇论文的方法部分就像做菜的食材配方和烹饪方法。如果读者看了方法后能够做出一样的菜肴,那说明方法写得恰当。方法部分将前言与结果部分联系起来,以创建清晰的故事线:我已经清晰告诉读者想做什么了,现在我要通过清晰的故事线告诉读者我准备如何做。

　　方法部分通常可以在研究开始时,甚至研究开始前就编写。

第 1 节　方法的内容

　　方法部分的目录可以用"Patients and methods"或"Methods"。副标题可根据需要进行扩展,以适应研究和目标期刊的要求。

　　如果在引言中提出了一个主要的研究问题和一个或多个次要问题,那么方法的描述从主要问题开始,然后是次要问题。

　　对于临床研究论文,如 RCT、病例对照研究或单臂研究,方法包括 6 个基本要素:研究设计、研究环境(Setting)、对象、干预方法、终点指标、数据收集和数据分析。这部分内容也可以参考"CONSORT 声明"。

　　研究设计一般包括研究类型(RCT? 还是非随机?)、何地、如何招募或选择研究对象、采用了哪些纳入/排除标准、数据测量方法和样本量计算方法。

　　数据测量方法包括检测时间和频率(例如,在筛查访视期间和 2 年随访期间,每月一次)。文献报道的检测方法如果是他人创建的,简单描述即可,但应引用原始研究文献。作者本人为研究而设计的方法要详细描写,如果很复杂,可以放在补充材料中。

　　对于治疗药物的报告,以下信息非常重要,写在正文中:

- 药物名称（化学、通用和品牌名称）；

- 剂量（以及对 BMI、血液学参数、肾功能或其他因素所做的任何调整）；

- 途径（如果是肠外途径，是否需要中心静脉通路?）；

- 静脉滴注的药物，需要描述稀释液的类型和体积，给药速率；

- 给药周期的长度和周期数，停药标准。

方法的描述要确保读者能够读懂，能够重复出来。

方法部分要声明该研究已得到独立的地方、区域或国家审查机构（例如伦理委员会）的批准，符合《赫尔辛基宣言》的要求，获得了知情同意（如果豁免，也要注明，包括豁免的理由）。有些杂志需要标注伦理批准号，如：

The study was conducted in accordance with the Declaration of Helsinki (as revised in 2013) and approved by institutional ethics committee of the hospital. Informed consent was obtained from all individual participants.

有些杂志要求显示本论文的撰写遵循"CONSORT 声明"，如：

We followed the Consolidated Standards of Reporting Trials (CONSORT) reporting guideline.

统计学方法的描述要详细，使有相应专业知识的读者能通过访问原始数据来判断该方法是否适合本研究，并核实所报告的结果。目前大牌的杂志编辑部也会有统计学专家参与审稿。具体介绍所使用的统计软件包及其版本。应区分事先设定的分析与探索性分析，包括亚组分析。

一般方法可按照以下副标题（Subheading）组织：

（1）患者（Subjects）：第一句说明研究的总体设计，如病例报告、病例系列、病例对照研究、队列研究和随机对照临床试验。指出数据收集是回顾性的还是前瞻性的。病例组和对照组是否随机选择；如果不是，他们是否代表某一人群？关于知情同意和机构审查委员会批准的声明也放此处。

中文论文习惯将患者的数量和年龄等信息放在方法中。这些信息只有研究开始后才知道，因此最好放在结果中。

（2）干预方法（Procedures）：在这一部分中，按照研究内容的时间顺序详细描述你做了什么。对于使用的主要设备，提供设备型号、制造商的名称和所在地，一般包括城市和国家。

（3）相关定义和标准（Definitions and criteria）：在本节中，应明确说明各种方法的定义和标准以及相关的参考文献。如果你设计了一个评分系统，那么每个类别的标准都应该明确说明。

（4）随访和数据收集（Data collection）：特别注意如何确保数据质量，如观察者内部和观察者之间的变异性评估。

（5）统计（Statistical analysis）：明确独立变量和因变量（结果）。样本大小和检验效能计算的声明也可以放在这段。本段最后一句应包括 P 值代表可接受的统计显著性水平的陈述。P 值一般为 0.05。如果选择了不同的级别（通常是更保守的级别），则应说明这一点并给出原因。

统计学方法不能太笼统，如：For statistical analysis, ANOVA test, chi-square test, T test, and Kruskal-Wallis test were used。应该具体描述每个数据对应的统计学方法，如：Chi-square tests were used in intergroup comparisons of categorical variables, and categorical variables were expressed as numbers, and percentages. In comparisons between cardiac failure rate, independent two samplest-test were used. In the evaluation of the factors effective on cardiac failure multivariate logistic regression test was used. P values lower than 0.05 were considered as statistically significant. The calculations were performed using a statistical package program (PASW v18, SPSS Inc, Chicago, IL).

我们还是以论文"A randomized trial of tai chi for fibromyalgia"为例介绍临床研究的方法描述[1]。

该文的方法部分一共有 7 个组成部分，分别是研究对象（Study participants）、研究设计（Study design）、太极干预方法（Tai Chi Intervention）、对照干预方法（Control intervention）、依从性（Adherence to programs）、结果和随访（Outcome measures and follow-up）和统计分析（Statistical analysis）。

第一部分"Study participants"，包括了研究的时间、地点、伦理批准、知情同意、入组标准、排除标准。

We conducted the trial from July 2007 through May 2009 at Tufts Medical Center, a tertiary care academic hospital in Boston. The institutional review board of the Tufts University Health Sciences Campus approved the study protocol. Eligible patients were 21 years of age or older and fulfilled the American College of Rheumatology 1990 diagnostic criteria for fibromyalgia. These criteria include a history of widespread musculoskeletal pain on the right and left sides of the body as well as above and below the waist, with a minimum duration of 3 months, and tenderness on pressure at 11 or more of 18 specific sites (tender points), with moderate or more severe tenderness reported on digital palpation.[16] We excluded persons who had participated in tai chi training within the past 6 months; those with serious medical conditions that might limit their participation; those with other diagnosed medical conditions known to contribute to fibromyalgia symptoms, such as thyroid disease, inflammatory arthritis, systemic lupus erythematosus, systemic sclerosis, rheumatoid arthritis, myositis, vasculitis, or Sjögren's syndrome; women who had a positive pregnancy test or who were planning to become pregnant during the study period; and persons who were unable to pass the Mini-Mental State Examination(i. e. , those with a score less than or equal to 24 [out of 30] points).[17] Participants were allowed to continue routine medications and maintain usual visits with their primary care physicians or rheumatologists throughout the study. All patients provided written informed consent.

我们于 2007 年 7 月至 2009 年 5 月在塔夫茨医学中心进行了这项试验，这是一家位于波士顿的三级教学医院。塔夫茨大学健康科学校区的机构审查委员会批准了研究方案。符合条件的患者为 21 岁或以上，符合美国风湿病学会 1990 年纤维肌痛诊断标准。这些标准包括身体右侧和左侧以及腰部上方和下方的广泛肌肉骨骼疼痛史，最短持续时间为 3 个月，以及 18 个特定部位(触痛点)中有 11 个或以上有压痛[16]；排除过去 6 个月内参加过太极训练的人；患有严重疾病可能限制其参与的人；患有已知会导致纤维肌痛症状的疾病的患者，如甲状腺疾病、炎性关节炎、系统性红斑狼疮、系统性硬化、类风湿性关节炎、肌炎、血管炎或干燥综合征；妊娠试验阳性或计划在研究期间怀孕的妇女[17]；在整个研究过程中参与者可继续常规药物治疗，并保持与初级保健医生或风湿病学专家的常规就诊。所有患者均签署书面知情同意书。

注意，方法中提到的诊断标准要提供参考文献。"三级教学医院"属于"Study setting"。

第二部分"Study design"，描述了具体的研究方法，包括如何分组、如何随机和如何保证盲法的实施。指出研究资助方没有参与研究的全过程(这部分可以不写)。资助方的资金支持放在致谢和在利益冲突部分说明。

We assigned participants to tai chi or the control intervention in three randomization cycles, using computer-generated numbers. The randomized treatment assignments were sealed in opaque envelopes and were opened individually for each patient who agreed to be in the study.

我们使用计算机生成的数字，将参与者分配到太极拳组或对照组。随机治疗分配数字被密封在不透明的信封中，每个同意参与研究的患者单独打开。

The sponsors had no role in the design and conduct of the study; the collection, management, analysis, or interpretation of the data; or the preparation, review, or approval of the manuscript. The study was conducted in accordance with the trial protocol.

资助方没有参与以下内容：研究的设计和实施；数据的收集、管理、分析或解释；或文稿的准备、审查或批准。研究按照试验方案进行。

第三部分"Tai Chi Intervention"，描述了太极拳治疗组的治疗方法。对于采用的杨氏太极拳提供了参考文献说明。

The tai chi intervention took place twice a week for 12 weeks, and each session lasted for 60 minutes. Classes were taught by a tai chi master with more than 20 years of teaching experience. In the first session, he explained the theory behind tai chi and its procedures and provided participants with printed materials on its principles and techniques. In subsequent sessions, participants practiced 10 forms from the classic Yang style of tai chi under his instruction[18]. Each session included a warm-up and self-massage, followed by a review of principles, movements, breathing techniques, and relaxation in tai chi. Throughout the intervention period, participants were instructed to practice tai chi at home for at least 20 minutes each day. At the end of the 12-week intervention, participants were encouraged to maintain their tai chi practice, using an instructional DVD, up until the follow-up visit at 24 weeks.

太极拳干预每周进行两次，为期 12 周，每次持续 60 分钟。课程由一位拥有 20 多年经验的太极师傅授课。第一节课太极师傅解释太极的理论及其动作，并向参与者提供了关于太极原理和技巧的印刷材料。在随后的课程中，参与者在他的指导下练习了经典杨式太极拳 10 式。每节课都包括热身、自我按摩以及复习太极拳的原理、动作、呼吸技巧和放松。在整个干预期间，要求参与者每天在家练习太极拳至少 20 分钟。在为期 12 周的干预结束时，鼓励参与者使用教学 DVD 保持太极练习，直到 24 周的随访。

第四部分"Control intervention"，描述了对照组是如何进行的。对于采用的对照方法提供了参考文献说明。

Our wellness education and stretching program similarly included 60-minute sessions held twice a week for 12 weeks[19]. At each session, a variety of health professionals provided a 40-minute didactic lesson on a topic relating to fibromyalgia, including the diagnostic criteria; coping strategies and problem-solving techniques; diet and nutrition; sleep disorders and fibromyalgia; pain management, therapies, and medications; physical and mental health; exercise; and wellness and lifestyle management[20]. For the final 20 minutes of each class, participants practiced stretching exercises supervised by the research staff. Stretches involved the upper body, trunk, and lower body and were held for 15 to 20 seconds. Participants were instructed to practice stretching at home for 20 minutes a day.

我们的健康教育和拉伸运动同样包括每周两次、为期 12 周的 60 分钟课程[19]。在每次课程中，健康专业人员都会就与纤维肌痛相关的主题提供 40 分钟的教学课程，包括诊断标准、应对策略和解决问题的技巧、饮食和营养、睡眠障碍和纤维肌痛、疼痛管理、疼痛治疗、疼痛药物、身心健康、运动以及健康和生活方式管理[20]。在每节课的最后 20 分钟，参与者在研究人员的指导下练习拉伸运动。拉伸包括上身、躯干和下身，并持续 15～20 秒。参与者被要求每天在家练习拉伸 20 分钟。

第五部分是"Adherence to programs"（遵守研究方案程度的监测）。

Participants in both groups were encouraged to continue their routine activities during the 12-week intervention period but were asked not to take part in any new, additional exercise programs. Adherence was maximized by an oral and written commitment from all participants at the baseline evaluation. The research staff asked participants who missed a class to attend a make-up class. Throughout the 12-week intervention period, we tracked the number of missed sessions and asked subjects to complete daily logs indicating the amount of time they practiced tai chi or stretching exercises.

鼓励两组的参与者都在 12 周的干预期内继续他们的日常活动，但要求他们不要参加任何新的、额外的锻炼计划。在基线评估时，要求参与者口头和书面承诺遵守研究方案，使他们的依从性达到最大。研究人员要求缺课的参与者参加补课。在为期 12 周的干预期间，我们跟踪了没有参与的训练次数，并要求受试者填写日志，记录他们练习太极拳或拉伸运动的时间。

第六部分"Outcome measures and follow-up"，描述了疗效指标和随访方法。一般来说疗效指标包括 1～2 个主要指标和多个次要指标。只有主要指标达到了预期的目的试验结果才能够被认为是有意义（Positive）。如果主要指标没有达到，则要在讨论部分重点讨论有差异的次要目标的临床价值，以"彰显"本研究的意义。

The primary outcome measure was the change in the Fibromyalgia Impact Questionnaire (FIQ) score from baseline to the end of the 12-week intervention. The FIQ is a well-validated, multidimensional measure of the overall severity of fibromyalgia as rated by patients. Categories include the intensity of pain, physical functioning, fatigue, morning tiredness, stiffness, depression, anxiety, job difficulty, and overall well-being[21]. The total score ranges from 0 to 100, with higher scores indicating more severe symptoms.

主要结果指标是从基线到 12 周干预结束时纤维肌痛影响问卷(FIQ)评分的变化。FIQ 是一个经过充分验证的多维度测量患者对纤维肌痛总体严重程度的方法,指标类别包括疼痛强度、身体机能、疲劳、晨间疲劳、僵硬、抑郁、焦虑、工作困难和总体健康状况[21]。总分范围从 0 到 100,分数越高表示症状越严重。

Secondary outcomes during the 12-week intervention included FIQ scores (obtained weekly). Global pain status was assessed separately by the participant and the study physician, who was unaware of the group assignment, with the use of a visual-analogue scale (VAS) (range, 0 to 10, with higher scores indicating greater pain). The study physician also determined the number of tender sites (of 18 sites in total) according to the standardized protocol[16,22]. The research staff, who were also unaware of the group assignments, evaluated participants' physical performance by measuring the time to completion of the 6-minute walk test (measured in yards)[23]. Additional measures included the score on the Pittsburgh Sleep Quality Index (PSQI) (range, 0 to 21, with higher scores indicating worse sleep quality)[24], the score on the depression scale of the Center for Epidemiologic Studies (CES-D) (range, 0 to 60, with higher scores indicating more severe depression)[25], the score on the Outcome Expectations for Exercise Scale (range, 1 to 5, with 1 indicating no expectations for exercise and 5 the highest expectations for exercise)[26], the score on the Chronic Pain Self-Efficacy Scale (CPSS) (range, 1 to 10, with higher scores indicating greater self-efficacy with respect to the management of chronic pain)[27], and the summary scores for the physical and mental quality-of-life components of the Medical Outcomes Study 36-Item Short-Form Health Survey (SF-36) (range, 0 to 100, with higher scores *indicating better health status*)[28].

12 周干预期间的次要结果包括 FIQ 分数(每周)。参与者和研究医生使用视觉模拟量表(VAS)(范围为 0~10 分,评分越高表示越疼)分别评估总体疼痛状态,采用盲法。研究医生还根据标准化方案确定了痛点的数量(共 18 个点)[16,22]。盲法下研究人员通过测量完成 6 分钟步行的距离(以码为单位)来评估参与者的身体表现[23]。其他措施包括匹兹堡睡眠质量指数(PSQI)评分(范围为 0~21 分,分越高表示睡眠质量越差)[24],流行病学研究中心(CES-D)抑郁量表评分(0~60 分,分越高表示抑郁越严重)[25],运动结果预期量表的分数(1~5 分,1 分表示不期望运动,5 分表示运动期望最高)[26],慢性疼痛自我效能表(CPSS)评分(范围为 1~10 分,分越高表示在慢性疼痛管理方面的自我能力感越高)[27],以及 SF-36 的身心生活质量部分的汇总分数(范围为 0 至 100,分越高表示健康状况越好)[28]。

Participants continued to take their regular medications, and we recorded any changes in the use of analgesics, antidepressants, anticonvulsants, muscle relaxants, benzodiazepines, dopamine agonists, or 5-hydroxytryptamine agonists. To test durability of the response, outcome measurements were repeated at the 24-week follow-up visit.

参与者继续服用常规药物,我们记录了镇痛药、抗抑郁药、抗惊厥药、肌肉松弛剂、苯二氮䓬类药物、多巴胺激动剂或 5-羟色胺激动剂的使用变化。为了评估太极疗效的持久性,在 24 周随访时结果指标将被重新评估。

Throughout the entire intervention period, we monitored adverse events, using a standard adverse-event case report form at each visit. This form included a description of all unanticipated benefits and undesirable experiences, particularly falls and exacerbations of fibromyalgia symptoms. Lack of an effect with tai chi or with stretching and wellness education was not considered an adverse event. By the nature of an exercise program, delayed muscle soreness (mild muscle pain or discomfort that occurred after exercise, did not require medical intervention, and resolved within 72 hours) was an expected outcome and thus was not considered an adverse event.

在整个干预期间,我们在每次就诊时使用标准的不良事件病例报告表监测不良事件。该表格包括所有未预料到的益处和不良体验的描述,特别是摔倒和纤维肌痛症状的加重。太极拳或拉伸和健康教育缺乏效果不被视为不良事件。根据运动的性质,延迟性肌肉酸痛(运动后出现的轻微肌肉疼痛或不适,不需要医疗干预,并在 72 小时内解决)是预期结果,因此不被视为不良事件。

注意,方法中提到的疗效评估标准要提供参考文献,而且由于《NEJM》是综合性杂志,读者来自不同的领域,对每个指标的分数高低和疾病程度的对应关系加以说明,以方便非本专业的读者理解。

一般不良反应应该单独一段。

第七部分"Statistical Analysis",描述了统计学方法和样本量计算方法。样本量计算方法也可以单独一段。

A trial conducted in Sweden, in which 58 participants were assigned to 32 weeks of either aquatic exercise or education (control), showed a significant effect size (i. e., standardized mean difference between groups) of 0.7 points in the FIQ score (mean [±SD] change, −0.9 ±1.3 in the exercise group vs. 0.0 ±1.4 in the control group)[29]. Guided by these results, we randomly assigned 66 patients to two groups (33 patients to each), which provided 78% power to detect a difference between means at a significance level of 5% with the use of a two-sided t-test.

在瑞典进行的一项试验中,58名参与者被分配到32周的水上运动或教育(对照组)中,结果显示FIQ评分的差异(即组间标准化平均差异)为0.7分(平均[±SD]变化,运动组为−0.9±1.3,对照组为0.0±1.4)[29]。根据这些结果,我们将66名患者随机分为两组(每组33名),使用双侧t检验,在显著性水平为5%的情况下,平均值之间的差异有78%的检测效能。

We compared between-group changes in outcomes at 0, 12, and 24 weeks (and weekly FIQ scores during the 12-week intervention) with mixed models … Effects were evaluated on an intention-to-treat basis, and participants who did not complete the follow-up period were considered not to have had any changes in scores. We tested for potential interactions between treatment and covariates, including age, sex, body-mass index, fibromyalgia duration, pain-severity score, coexisting illnesses, health status, and medication use. A two-sided P value of less than 0.05 indicated statistical significance. Results are presented as between-group differences with 95% confidence intervals.

我们使用混合模型比较0周、12周和24周的组间结果变化(以及12周干预期间的每周FIQ得分)……在意向治疗的基础上评估效果,未完成随访的参与者被认为得分没有任何变化。我们评估了治疗与协变量之间的潜在相互作用,包括年龄、性别、体重指数、纤维肌痛持续时间、疼痛严重程度评分、共病、健康状况和药物使用。双侧P值小于0.05表明有统计学意义。结果采用 95% 置信区间的组间差异来标示。

研究方法部分采用过去时, 尽量采用主动语态。

第 2 节 方法部分注意事项

"Try" "use" "perform" 和 "make" 常常会隐藏真正的动作词, 如 "a needle valve was used to regulate pressure" 应当写成 "a needle valve regulated pressure", 因为重点是 "regulate pressure", 不是 "use a needle valve"。

在统计部分, 注意统计的实施用过去时, 但统计结果的展现方法的描述用现在时, 如:

> Effects <u>were evaluated</u> on an intention-to-treat basis. Continuous variables were summarized with means and standard deviations (if normally distributed) and medians and interquartile ranges (if positively skewed). Results <u>are presented</u> as between-group differences with 95% confidence intervals. Outcome analyses <u>are reported</u> with 95% confidence intervals.

在起草了方法部分之后, 问问自己:"读者能用我提供的信息重现我们的研究吗?"

第 3 节 补充文件

有些研究方法很复杂, 治疗方案的信息非常重要, 但文字可能会超过版面的字数限定。这时, 有些方法可以写在补充文件上 (Supplementary file)。

第 4 节 高通量研究的数据

一般杂志要求作者将他们的高通量数据, 包括 mRNA、miRNA、蛋白质组学和基因组 DNA (arrayCGH、芯片和 SNP) 阵列存储到公共数据库中, 如 Gene Expression Omnibus (GEO) 或 Array Express, 或作者自己的开放数据库。方法部分必须提供一个登录号或网站链接, 带有有效的访问代码。

第 5 节　数据共享声明

大部分杂志要求作者必须向其他研究人员提供原始数据，在方法部分末尾包含一个标题为"数据共享声明"的小节。本小节应包括有关如何访问数据库的信息：

➤ For original data, please contact name@example.org.

➤ Microarray data are available at GEO under accession number ×××××××××.

➤ X data may be found in a data supplement available with the online version of this article. Y data have been deposited to www.example.org.

ICMJE 的指南要求临床试验论文必须说明是否可以共享去身份信息(deidentified)的参与者的数据，声明应包括以下信息：

• 是否会共享去身份信息的参与者数据。

• 哪些特定数据和文档将被共享。

• 共享数据的方法和截止时间。

• 访问数据所需的条件(如有)。

例句：

➤ Deidentified individual participant data are available indefinitely at www.example.org. The study protocol, analytic code …［etc.］ are also available at the same website.

➤ Deidentified individual participant data that underlie the reported results will be made available 3 months after publication for a period of 5 years after the publication date at www.example.org. Proposals for access should be sent to name@example.org.

➤ Individual participant data will not be shared.

参考文献

[1] Wang C, Schmid C H, Rones R, et al. A randomized trial of tai chi for fibromyalgia. N Engl J Med. 2010,363(8):743 – 754.

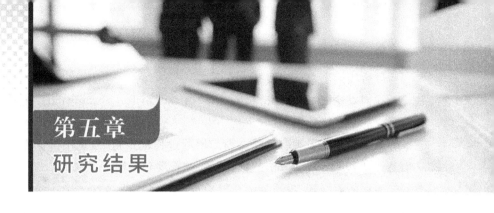

结果部分是论文的主要部分。结果的描述要做到以下几点：

1. 主次分明。临床研究的结果描述和基础研究不一样，除了先描述参与者的基线资料外，接下来是主要疗效结果，其次是次要结果。而基础研究一般按照先后发现的顺序描述。

2. 描述要清晰简洁，为此结果部分要充分利用图和表格。

3. 结果和方法要一一对应：对于每个方法，都应该有相应的结果（发现），反之亦然。如果在方法部分中使用了副标题，那么在结果部分中尽量以相同的顺序提供相同的副标题。如果方法和结果都没有副标题，两者的布局尽量一致。

4. 副标题尽量用短语。如果用句子，一般用现在时。

第 1 节　结果的一般组成

临床研究的结果常见顺序是：研究对象的招募情况、基线特征、主要结果、次要结果和不良反应（并发症）。

结果部分的第一部分应描述研究人群的基本特征。RCT 论文首先要提供招募程序流程图，通常是论文的图 1。下一步是描述研究样本的特征，如每组患者数量、性别比例、年龄分布以及和研究结果可能相关的主要临床和生活方式变量，通常为论文的表 1。数据一般用均值和标准差，或中值和范围的形式报告。基线比较的目的是让读者知道干预组和对照组是否相似。

中文文章习惯把研究样本的特征，如年龄、性别和数量放在方法中，这是不符合逻辑的。因为方法属于研究计划，而年龄和性别的比例是在研究开始后才知道的，因此属于结果。

第二部分描述疗效。应按照方法部分所述的相同顺序报告各项结果。

最后描述不良反应或并发症。

我们以论文"A randomized trial of tai chi for fibromyalgia"为例介绍临床研究的结果描述[1]。

第一段描述了患者招募过程。招募过程也很重要，从中可以看出招募的难易程度和患者对新方法的信任度。此段要包括时间和地点：

Between July 2007 and December 2008, we screened 356 patients by telephone. Of the 124 patients who resided near Boston, 90 qualified for the baseline evaluation; 24 patients in this group were excluded for various reasons, and the 66 eligible participants were randomly assigned in equal numbers to either the tai chi intervention or the control intervention (Fig.1).

2007 年 7 月至 2008 年 12 月，我们通过电话筛查了 356 名患者。在波士顿附近的 124 名患者中有 90 人符合基线评估标准；有 24 名患者因各种原因被排除在外，66 名符合条件的参与者被随机分配到同等数量的太极拳干预组或对照干预组（图 1）。

第二段描述了患者干预之前的基线情况，理论上随机分配后组间的各个指标的相似的，不应该存在统计学有意义的差异。如果有差异，要对结果进行校正分析（Adjusted）。这部分内容通过表格来显示，一目了然。正文中只描述最重要的参数，如年龄和病程，其他则放在表格中：

Table 1 shows baseline data for the 66 participants before randomization. Participants had a mean age of 50 years, 86% were women, and 56% were white, the mean body-mass index (the weight in kilograms divided by the square of the height in meters) was 32.7. On average, participants had had fibromyalgia for 11 years. Baseline characteristics were reasonably well balanced between the two groups, except that the tai chi group had a lower CES-D score. The average score on the physical component of the SF-36 was about 2 SD below normal, indicating a cohort with poor health.

表 1 显示了随机分组前 66 名参与者的基线数据。参与者的平均年龄为 50 岁，86% 为女性，56% 为白人，平均体重指数为 32.7。参与者纤维肌痛平均时间 11 年。除了太极组的 CES-D 评分较低外，两组的基线特征相当均衡。SF-36 身体部分的平均得分比正常值低约 2 SD，表明该人群健康状况不佳。

第三段是两组的依从性比较。依从性数据也可以放在结果的最后。

The rate of attendance during the 12-week intervention was 77% for the tai chi group and 70% for the control group. Five patients withdrew from the study by 12 weeks, and seven by 24 weeks (Fig. 1).

12 周干预期间,太极组的参与率为 77%,对照组为 70%。5 名患者在 12 周后退出研究,7 名患者在 24 周后退出(图 1)。

第四至九段采用图、表和文字结合的方法描述主要指标,即 FIQ 分数。文字描述了主要结果,即 12 周和 24 周的 FIQ 数值和组间差异,以及 12 周的其他指标的差异。24 周的其他指标的差异则只做总结,不再赘述具体数值。

Table 2 and Figure 2 show changes from baseline to 12 and 24 weeks in the two groups for all outcomes.

表 2 和图 2 显示了两组从基线到 12 周和 24 周的所有结果的变化。

At 12 weeks, the tai chi group had a significantly greater decrease in the total FIQ score than did the control group (-27.8 points [95% confidence interval {CI}, -33.8 to -21.8] vs. -9.4 points [95% CI, -15.5 to -3.4]). The mean between-group difference was -18.4 points (95% CI, -26.9 to -9.8). Figure 3 shows that the mean between-group difference in FIQ scores gradually increased during the intervention. Similarly, at 24 weeks the tai chi group had a significant reduction in symptoms (change in the total FIQ score from baseline to 24 weeks, -28.6 points [95% CI, -34.8 to -22.4]), which was greater than the improvement in the control group; the mean between-group difference in the change from baseline to 24 weeks was -18.3 points (95% CI, -27.1 to -9.6; P<0.001).

在 12 周时,太极组的 FIQ 总分下降幅度明显大于对照组{-27.8 分[95% CI(CI),-33.8 至-21.8],对照组是-9.4 分[95% CI,-15.5 至-3.4]}。组间平均差异为-18.4 分(95% CI,-26.9 至-9.8)。图 3 显示,干预期间,FIQ 得分的组间平均差异逐渐增加。同样,在 24 周时,太极拳组症状显著减少[FIQ 总分从基线到 24 周的变化为-28.6 分(95% CI,-34.8 至-22.4)],这比对照组的改善更大;从基线到 24 周变化的组间平均差异为 -18.3 分(95% CI,-27.1 至-9.6;P<0.001)。

At 12 weeks, the tai chi group had greater mean improvement in sleep quality than the control group, as measured by the change in the PSQI score (mean between-group difference, -2.9 points [95% CI, -4.6 to -1.2]; P=0.001) …. The change from baseline to 12 weeks in the physician's objective global assessment also differed significantly between the two groups (mean between-group difference, -1.1 points [95% CI, -1.9 to -0.2]; P=0.02). The 6-minute walk test was significantly better with tai chi at 12 weeks (mean between-group difference, 44.4 yd [95% CI, 12.3 to 76.4]; $P=0.007$). At 12 weeks, the tai chi group also had greater improvement in the scores for the SF-36 physical component(mean between-group difference, 7.1 points [95% CI, 3.1 to 11.1]; $P=0.001$), the SF-36 mental component (mean between-group difference, 6.1 points [95% CI, 0.7 to 11.6]; $P=0.03$), and the CES-D(mean between-group difference, −5.9 points [95% CI, −9.8 to −1.9]; $P=0.005$). The tai chi group had greater improvement in the CPSS score, but the difference was not significant(mean between-group difference, 1.0 point [95% CI, −0.03 to 2.0]; $P=0.06$). The body-mass index remained stable in both groups

在 12 周时,太极组的睡眠质量平均改善程度高于对照组,这是通过 PSQI 评分的变化来衡量的(组间平均差异,−2.9 分[95% CI,−4.6 至−1.2]; $P=0.001$)……医生客观总体评估从基线到 12 周的变化在两组之间也有显著差异(组间差异,−1.1 分[95% CI,−1.9 至−0.2]; $P=0.02$)。12 周时,6 分钟步行测试太极拳组明显有优势(组间平均差异为 44.4 码[95% CI,12.3 至 76.4]; $P=0.007$)。12 周时,太极拳组在 SF-36 身体成分得分方面也有较大改善(组间差异为 7.1 分[95% CI,3.1 至 11.1]; $P=0.001$),SF-36 心理成分(组间平均差异,6.1 分[95% CI,0.7 至 11.6]; $P=0.03$)和 CES-D(组间差异,−5.9 分[95% CI,−9.8 至−1.9]; $P=0.005$),但差异不显著(组间平均差异,1 分[95% CI,−0.03 至 2.0]; $P=0.06$)。两组的体重指数保持稳定。

Improvements with tai chi were maintained at 24 weeks for sleep quality, the patients' and physicians' global assessments, the scores for the SF-36 physical and mental components, and the CES-D score. The changes from baseline to 24 weeks in the 6-minute walk test and the CPSS score also favored tai chi over the control intervention, but the between-group difference was not significant.

在睡眠质量、患者和医生的总体评估、SF-36 身体和心理部分的评分以及 CES-D 评分方面,太极组的改善在 24 周还很明显。在 6 分钟步行测试中,从基线到 24 周的变化以及 CPSS 评分太极组也比对照组更倾向于好转,但组间差异并不显著。

Table 3 shows that, with a clinically meaningful change in the FIQ score defined as 8.1 points, 30 significantly more patients in the tai chi group than in the control group had improvement: 79% versus 39%($P=0.001$) at 12 weeks, and 82% versus 53%($P=0.009$) at 24 weeks. The tai *chi group also met standards for clinically meaningful improvement in the patient's VAS score for pain and in sleep-quality, CES-D, and SF-36 scores significantly more often than did controls (Table 3).*

表 3 显示,如果 FIQ 评分的临床意义变化被定义为 8.1 分,太极组有 30 名患者发生变化,明显多于对照组:12 周时分别是 79% 和 39% (P=0.001),24 周时分别是 82% 和 53% (P=0.009)。太极组在患者疼痛 VAS 评分、睡眠质量、CES-D 和 SF-36 评分方面达到临床有意义的病人比例显著高于对照组 (表 3)。

All treatment effects remained significant after adjusting for the baseline CES-D score, and no interactions with treatment were found. No adverse events were noted during the study interventions.

调整基线 CES-D 评分后,所有治疗效果仍然显著,未发现会影响治疗。研究干预期间未发现不良事件。

最后一段是对对症用药的比较:

At 12 weeks, more subjects had discontinued medication used to treat fibromyalgia in the tai chi group than in the control group, but the difference was not significant (11 of 31 patients vs. 4 of 26, P=0.09).

在 12 周时,太极组中停用治疗纤维肌痛药物的受试者多于对照组,但差异不显著(分别是 31 例患者中有 11 例,26 例患者中有 4 例,P=0.09)。

第 2 节 描述结果时的注意事项

一般的论文结果部分仅用于报告事实和数字,相关解释放在讨论部分。但也有些杂志将结果和讨论合并。这时候每个结果后面可以进行相应的讨论。

确保单位和数字正确。当数字不对或不合理时,论文几乎会被拒稿。

有些结果的临床意义读者都看得明白,如治疗组舒张压降到 80 mmHg,对照组降到 95 mmHg,治疗的价值显然易见。对于读者可能不大了解的指标,应说明结果是否具有临床意义,而不是仅仅有统计学意义。统计意义是证据强度的陈述,不一定具有临床重要性。如:*The tai chi group also met standards for clinically meaningful improvement in the patients' VAS score.*

有些结果可以在讨论中介绍,并用"data not shown"说明。

结果部分是文字、图和表格之间的动态交互。图和表对于显示大量数据特别有用。尽量使用表格和图表来体现结果。文字通常只描述表格和图表中的重要信息，不要重复全部信息。重要信息指支持研究假设的数据、意外的发现和严重不良反应。

有些杂志建议：如果要报告统计学处理的结果差异，最好使用"statistically significant"，不要单独用"significant"，以免和临床疗效的显著差异混淆。

对于没有显著差异，但又有一些差异的结果，为了表明确实有差异，可以这样描述：

➢ Although not statistically significant, the median survival time for the experimental arm <u>was numerically superior</u> to the control arm.

➢ Although not statistically significant, the median survival time for the experimental arm <u>tended to be longer</u> than that of the control arm.

➢ The changes from baseline to 24 weeks in the 6-minute walk test <u>favored tai chi over</u> the control intervention, but the between-group difference was not significant.

➢ At 12 weeks, more subjects had discontinued medication used to treat fibromyalgia in the tai chi group than in the control group, but the difference was not significant(11 of 31 patients vs. 4 of 26, $P=0.09$).

除了均值和 P 值外，疗效指标要加上 95% 置信区间。95% 置信区间显示了治疗效果的方向及其精确度。

避免使用"remarkably"或"strikingly"等词语。

灵活使用不同句式来呈现结果，如：

At 12 weeks, the tai chi group had a significantly greater decrease in the total FIQ score than did the control group.

Similarly, at 24 weeks the tai chi group had a significant reduction in symptoms, which was greater than the improvement in the control group.

At 12 weeks, the tai chi group had greater mean improvement in sleep quality than the control group.

The change from baseline to 12 weeks in the physicians' objective global assessment also differed significantly between the two groups(mean between-group difference, −1.1 points; $P=0.02$).

The 6-minute walk test was significantly better with tai chi at 12 weeks (mean between-group difference, 44.4 yd; $P=0.007$).

At 12 weeks, the tai chi group also had greater improvement in the scores for the SF-36 physical component(mean between-group difference,

7. 1 points；P＝0. 001）and the CES-D（mean between-group difference，
-5. 9 points；P＝0. 005）.

Table 3 shows that，with a clinically meaningful change in the FIQ
score defined as 8. 1 points，significantly more patients in the tai chi group
than in the control group had improvement：79％ versus 39％（P＝0. 001）
at 12 weeks，and 82％ versus 53％（P＝0. 009）at 24 weeks.

The tai chi group also met standards for clinically meaningful
improvement in the patient's VAS score for pain significantly more often
than did controls.

包含多个组的研究，呈现数据时始终使用相同的顺序，一般先描写试验组的结果，再描写对照组的结果。对应地，在表格中，左边是试验组，右边是对照组。

两组间有多个数据要比较时，如果多个指标在治疗组有进步，可以用"in favor of"，而用比较级反而不方便：

Differences in favor of vedolizumab over placebo were also seen with
respect to mPDAI-defined remission at week 34（difference，17％；95％ CI，
0 to 35），mPDAI-defined response at week 14（difference，30％；95％ CI，
8 to 48）and at week 34（difference，22％；95％ CI，2 to 40），and PDAI-
defined remission at week 14（difference，25％；95％ CI，8 to 41）and at
week 34（difference，19％；95％ CI，2 to 37）.

数字使用有临床意义的小数，如对于血压值，小数点后面一位即可。

描写效果的时候，百分比数字后面一定要有绝对数字。例如，"The percentage was 20％（2/10）in the intervention group compared with 10％ （1/10）in the control group"。这样做的意义很明显，同样的百分比，如果病例数不一样，可信度差异很大。如同样是 10％ 的治愈率，10 个患者有 1 个治愈和 1000 个患者有 100 个治愈的研究，显然可信度不一样。

有些杂志要求小于 0. 001 的 P 值报告为 $P＜0. 001$；对于 $0. 001＜P＜0. 01$，则写出具体的 3 位数，如 $P＝0. 004$；对于 $0. 01＜P＜0. 1$，写具体 2 位数，如 $P＝0. 05$；对于 $0. 1＜P＜0. 9$，写具体 1 位数，如 $P＝0. 6$；对于 $P＞0. 9$，写 $P＞0. 9$ 即可。

研究结果中一般不写方法。但有时候为了让读者可以通过快速阅读结果了解全文；或者方法太多，为了方便读者能够把方法和结果一一对应，有些作者在结果中会简单描述方法。这种风格在基础研究中用得比较多。如下面的例子中，因为有 3 个不同的实验部分，为了避免混淆，每次结果的描述都会简单叙述方法[2]：

In the first set of experiments, we randomized 64 rats to either the M-CLP group or the CLP group. After operation, 19 rats survived in the M-CLP group and 26 in the CLP group. All surviving rats were sacrificed at 24 hours. Blood samples were collected for organ function evaluation. Of the 19 rats in the M-CLP group, 17 met the SEPSIS 3.0 criteria. Of the 26 rats in the CLP group, only 7 met the SEPSIS 3.0 criteria. Thus, more rats in the M-CLP group developed sepsis than did rats in the traditional CLP group 24 hours postoperatively (53.1% vs 21.9%, P=0.01).

在第一组实验中,我们将 64 只大鼠随机分为 M-CLP 组或 CLP 组。术后,M-CLP 组 19 只大鼠存活,CLP 组 26 只大鼠生存。24 小时处死所有存活的大鼠。采集血样用于器官功能评估。在 M-CLP 组的 19 只大鼠中,17 只符合 SEPSIS 3.0 标准。CLP 组 26 只大鼠中,只有 7 只符合 SEPSIS 3.0 标准。因此,术后 24 小时,M-CLP 组的大鼠比传统 CLP 组更常发生脓毒血症(53.1%对 21.9%,P=0.01)。)

又如:

We set out to identify drug targets that may help restore defective lung repair. To achieve this, we used a transcriptomics-guided target discovery strategy (described in Fig.1A) based on gene signatures of COPD lung tissues (8) and of a model of CS exposure (9) to identify differentially regulated druggable genes. We found reactome pathways related to inflammation such as neutrophil degranulation and innate immune system to be enriched in both datasets (Fig.1, C and D) and pathways related senescence, apoptosis, and extracellular matrix regulation to be enriched in COPD, which was also reported in a recent study (7) using longitudinal samples.

我们计划寻找可能有助于恢复肺修复能力缺陷的药物靶点。为了实现这一点,我们使用转录组学指导的靶点发现策略(如图 1A 所示)。该策略基于 COPD 肺组织(8)和 CS 暴露模型(9)的基因特征,以识别差异调节的、可作为药物靶点的基因。我们发现,与炎症相关的反应通路(如中性粒细胞脱颗粒和先天免疫系统)在两个数据集中都有富集(图 1,C 和 D),与衰老、凋亡和细胞外基质调节相关的通路则在 COPD 中有富集,这也在最近的一项使用纵向样本的研究(7)中有发现。

第 3 节 图

表格和图表是展示研究数据很好的方式。如果设计得好，它们所提供的信息比用语言表达的要多。一篇论文的大部分结果应该以表格和图表的形式呈现，因为读者将通过表格和图表能够快速了解研究的全貌。

如果要显示不同类别中变量的数量或百分比，使用条形图（Bar chart）或直方图（Histogram）比较好。

条形图，又称柱形图，是一种以长方形的长度为变量的图，用来比较两个或以上的价值（不同时间或者不同条件）。长条图亦可横向排列，或用多维方式表达。根据数据内容，条形图的表现方式可以灵活多样。如，为了表示Inhibitor 1 对 Substance A，B 和 C 的合成的抑制作用，可以采用图 5.1。

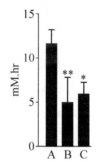

图 5.1　**Production of A，B，and C in the presence of inhibitor 1（1mM）after 24h of fermentation．* denotes vs Substance A．* $P<0.05$，* * $P<0.01$．**

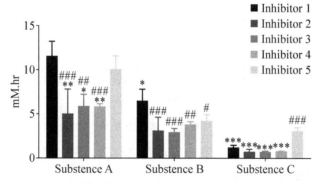

图 5.2　**Production of A，B，and C in the presence of inhibitors 1，2，3，4，and 5（1mM） after 24 h of fermentation．# denotes vs Inhibitor 1 and * denotes vs Inhibitor 5．*，# $P<0.05$，* *，# # $P<0.01$，* * *，# # # $P<0.001$．**

如果我们想表示 5 个"Inhibitor"对 A、B 和 C 的合成的抑制作用，可以采用图 5.2。

直方图一般用横轴表示数据类型，纵轴表示数据值。直方图也可以被归一化以显示"相对"频率，其高度等于 1。

如果对一组受试者的两个数值测量值进行比较，则选散点图（Scatter plot）。如图 5.3 为一组研究对象的身高和体重的分布。

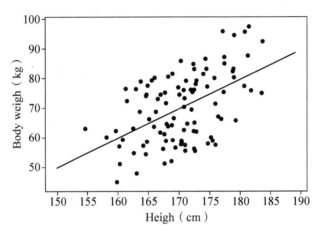

图 5.3　散点图

折线图（Line chart）可用于显示定量变量随时间的变化，如不同月份卧床老人摔倒的次数（图 5.4）。

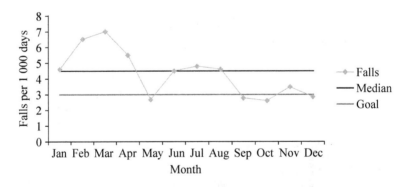

图 5.4　折线图

饼图（Pie chart）最好用于显示资源信息，例如属于各种类别的人口的相对比例或百分比（图 5.5）。

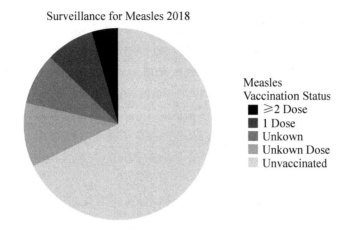

Surveillance for Measles 2018

Measles
Vaccination Status
■ ≥2 Dose
■ 1 Dose
■ Unkown
■ Unkown Dose
□ Unvaccinated

图 5.5　饼图

有些杂志初次提交时不要求使用高分辨率图像文件,因为高分辨率图像不方便上传。论文接受后可再提供高分辨率的图。

需要注意的是,不能对一张图像中的任何部分进行调节,包括增强、模糊、移动、删除或加入。如果使用了来自同一凝胶或显微镜视野下的不同部分的图像,或来自不同凝胶、视野的图像,则必须通过图形的排列(即插入黑色分界线)和文字说明来明确这些图像是组合的。

对整个图像的亮度、对比度或颜色平衡的调整是允许的,但前提是不能模糊、消除或歪曲原始图像中的任何信息,包括背景。非线性调整必须在图例中说明。除非绝对必要,不要使用图像编辑软件中提供的特殊软件工具(如擦除),如果有此类操作都必须在图例中予以解释。

有印刷版的期刊(主要是那些老牌杂志),彩图要收费,按照有彩图的页数的数量收,而不是按照图的数量,大约每页收 600 美元,因此如果没有必要的话,就用黑白或灰度图,但要确保打印后清晰。通常这些杂志的网络版发表彩图是免费的。因此作者可以选择网络版用彩图,印刷版用黑白图。

只有网络版的杂志不额外收彩图费。

为了尽量利用空间,一般图的宽度应该布满 1 列或 2 列。高度则没有上、下限。作者应确保图像的所有部分彼此成比例,符合审美标准。

图例(Text legend)包括编号(如 Figure 1)和标题,一般用粗体。标题最好用短语,之后是非粗体的内容描述。如:

➢ **Figure 4. Clusters of genes categorized by the expression patterns in different cells.** The vertical axis represents the normalized gene expression values. (A) Representative genes that were predominantly expressed in A cells. (B) Representative genes that were up-regulated in B cells. (C) Representative genes that were highly expressed in C cells.

图例的标题如果用句子,一般用现在时。描述部分用过去时,如:

➤ **Fig. 1 | NK cells from patients with severe COVID-19 fail to control virus replication.** Vero E6 cells(a) or Calu-3 cells(b) were infected with SARS-CoV-2(B. 1 lineage). At 1 h after infection, NK cells from healthy donors activated for 24 h in vitro as indicated with interleukins were added. Viral replication was measured 12 h later as genome equivalents(GE) per ml (GE ml^{-1})

如果一个图形仅包含 2 个或 3 个组,有些杂志不建议用字母标记,而是建议用"top", "bottom", "left", "right"和"middle panels",如:

➤ **Figure 1. Cyclin D1 immunostaining of cell nuclei.** Shown at ×20 original magnification(left) and×400 original magnification(right).

➤ **Figure 1. Cyclin D1 immunostaining of cell nuclei.** (Left) ×20 original magnification. (Right) ×400 original magnification.

图例中会常常使用缩写。缩写应在图例中说明。注意,"control"的缩写是"Ctrl",不是"con"。

图中的不同组可以用图标说明:

➤ Symbols represent treatment groups($n=4$ rats/group):saline(•), 0. 4 g/kg(■), 1 g/kg(▲), and 2 g/kg(♦).

➤ Symbols represent treatment groups($n=4$ rats/group):• indicates saline;■, 0. 4 g/kg;▲, 1 g/kg; and ♦, 2 g/kg.

或者用文字说明图中的符号,如:

➤ Cells were incubated with 1 000 ng/mL IL-2(triangles) or IL-6(squares) in plates containing 0(open symbols) or 500(filled symbols) μg/mL aspirin.

图例中包括统计显著性水平的标识(通常用星号标记:$^* P<0.05$,$^{**} P<0.01$,$^{***} P<0.001$)。

对于图中的每张显微照片(无论是显微照片还是电子显微照片,包括inset),应注明放大倍数。这可以通过在显微照片图像中包含比例尺(scale bar)或在图例中说明显微照片的原始放大率来实现,如"Bars represent 5 μm (A) and 200 nm(C)"。放大倍数也可这样描述:"Original magnification × 250;Original magnification × 250 for all panels;Original magnifications × 250(A-D) and ×400(E-H)."

Inset 是一个图中的局部放大部分。Inset 的意思如果从图中一目了然的话,可以不在图例中解释,如图5.6。

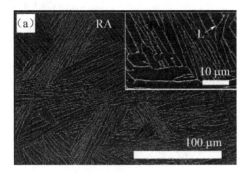

图 5.6 局部放大图示例

第 4 节 表 格

表格通常至少有六个元素:① 表格编号,② 表格标题,③ 行标题
(stubs),④ 列标题(boxes),⑤ 数据,以及⑥ 水平线(rules)。大多数表中还
有脚注、行副标题,以及缩写的全称,如表5.1。

Table 5.1   Baseline Characteristics of the Study Participants.[*]

Variable	Tai Chi Group (N=33)	Control Group (N=33)
Female sex-no. of patients(%)	28(85)	29(88)
Age-yr	49.7 ± 11.8	50.5 ± 10.5
White race-no. of patients(%)[†]	20(61)	17(52)
High-school or higher education-no. of patients(%)	31(94)	30(91)
Body-mass index[‡]	33.9 ± 8.9	31.5 ± 7.4
Duration of fibromyalgia-related pain-yr	11.8 ± 6.9	10.0 ± 7.2
Medications taken before intervention-no. of patients(%)		
Analgesics	29(88)	24(73)
Antidepressants	17(51)	15(45)
Anticonvulsants	9(27)	5(15)

Variable	Tai Chi Group (N=33)	Control Group (N=33)
Muscle relaxants	9(27)	4(12)
Benzodiazepines	5(15)	3(9)
Self-reported coexisting illness-no. of patients(%)		
Heart disease	0	0
Hypertension	12(36)	6(18)
Diabetes	6(18)	1(3)
FIQ score[§]	62.9±15.5	68.0±11
Visual-analogue scale[¶]		
Patient's global assessment	5.8±2.3	6.3±1.8
Physician's global assessment	5.7±1.9	5.6±2.4
PSQI score[‖]	13.9±3.1	13.5±3.7
SF-36 score[**]		
Physical component	28.5±8.4	28.0±7.8
Mental component	42.6±12.2	37.8±10.5
CES-D score[††]	22.6±9.2	27.8±9.2
CPSS score[‡‡]	5.2±1.9	4.6±2.2
6-Minute walk test-yd[§§]	522.1±102.7	501.2±106.6
Outcome Expectations for Exercise score[¶¶]	3.7±0.8	3.9±0.7

* Plus-minus values are means ±SD unless otherwise noted.

†Race was reported by the patients.

‡The body-mass index is the weight in kilograms divided by the square of the height in meters. This value was missing for one patient in the tai chi group.

§ The Fibromyalgia Impact Questionnaire (FIQ) assesses physical function, common symptoms, and general well-being in fibromyalgia. Scores range from 0 to 100, with higher scores indicating more severe symptoms.

¶ Patient global status was assessed separately by the participant and the study physician with the use of a visual-analogue scale. Scores range from 0 to 10, with 0 equaling no pain.

‖ Scores on the Pittsburgh Sleep Quality Index (PSQI) range from 0 to 21, with higher scores indicating worse sleep quality.

∗∗ The Medical Outcomes Study 36-Item Short-Form Health Survey (SF-36) is a self-administered, 36-item questionnaire that assesses the concepts of physical functioning, role limitations due to physical problems, social function, bodily pain, general mental health, role limitations due to emotional problems, vitality, and general health perceptions. Note that both the physical and mental component summaries can be combined. Scores range from 0 to 100, with higher scores indicating better health status.

†† Scores on the Center for Epidemiologic Studies Depression (CES-D) index range from 0 to 60, with higher scores indicating more dysphoria. The difference between the scores of the two treatment groups was significant ($P < 0.05$).

‡‡ The Chronic Pain Self-Efficacy Scale (CPSS) reflects the patients' confidence in their ability to perform a particular behavior or task and is believed to be a determinant of fibromyalgia symptoms. Scores range from 1 to 10, with higher scores indicating better status.

§§ The 6-minute walk test measures the distance covered during the 6-minute walk (in yards) as an objective assessment of mobility. It was considered to be a proxy for physical function, with higher scores indicating improved functional conditioning in fibromyalgia. To convert yards to meters, multiply by 0.914 4.

¶¶ Scores on the Outcome Expectations for Exercise Scale range from 1 to 5, with higher scores indicating high outcome expectations.

该表格具有典型的英文论文表格特征：

• 三线表。

• 第一行参数，英文是"Item""Variable"。各参数首字母大写。

• 第一栏各干预组的患者数量要显示。

• 某个参数如果有二级参数，二级参数的首个字母缩进，如"Medications

taken before intervention"参数下有"Analgesics""Antidepressants"等二级参数。

• 《NEJM》的表格下的脚注比较详细，主要是为了方便读者通过表格就能够读懂文章的主要结果，但一般杂志不这样做。脚注中关于常识的介绍用现在时，研究数据的介绍用过去时。

• 性别只显示女性，男性不必写。

表格标题一般用短语。

通常，表格中比较的两个（或以上）的组别应该并排进行，而不是上下排列。最后一列可显示研究组之间比较的 P 值。如果随机临床试验的基线各组是均衡的，不写 P 值。

一般从左到右进行比较（左边干预组，右边对照组）。

栏目的标题尽量不要用模糊的代号，例如 A 组、B 组、C 组等。

列标题和行标题应该包括组的样本量和度量单位。表格一般采用无边界网格，没有垂直线和尽量少的水平线（典型的三线表）。表格的第一列通常是变量（Variables 或 Items）。变量的度量单位可以放在正下方的括号中。如果整个表格只有一个度量单位，则放在标题中。

表格的列的标题要简短（最多两行）。表格中行和列标题的首字母应大写。

有些杂志要求表格的行或列标题或表标题中不使用">""<"">"和"<"，要求使用短语，如：

➢ Less than 200 mg（不用<200 mg）

➢ Older than 60 years（不用>60 years）

➢ At least 60 years old（不用>60 years）

➢ At least 1 year old（不用>1 year）

➢ 2 or more treatments（不用>2 treatments）

➢ Platelet count no higher than 100×10^9/L（不用 Platelet count < 100×10^9/L）

脚注如果有多个省略词汇，要用并列句，不要重复使用 indicates，可用逗号代替，如："BM indicates bone marrow; SCT, stem cell transplantation; and VWF, von Willebrand factor"。

表格的单元格（cells）包含数字、文字或符号。每个单元都必须包含信息；如果没有可用信息，可以使用"NA""－"或"n/a"，并在脚注中将其定义为不可用或不适用（not available or not applicable）。

列的内容需要对齐；单词通常是左对齐的，数字则以小数点、括号或 10^n

对齐。

表格脚注应简短,并提供缩写和统计学符号。有时候要解释数据差异,例如,"由于四舍五入,百分数的合计不是100"（percentages do not total 100 because of rounding）。

第5节 图表应该注意的问题

图表必须是不言自明的（Self-explanatory）,即读者可以不阅读正文的内容就能完全理解图表所需表达的意思。

一般来说,容易用语言表达的简单的结果就不要用图和表。

一定要仔细设计表格和图表的布局,这对于审稿过程也是至关重要的。混乱的图表会让编辑和审稿人花费时间去理解,从而降低被接受的概率。使用专用软件制作图形可以提高图形质量。

印刷版的期刊图和表加起来一般只允许6个。额外的图表常可以作为补充材料放在杂志的网站供读者下载。也可以把多个逻辑上、内容上关联的图合并为一个图。

正文的文字应避免重复图表中的所有信息,文字主要强调图表中支持自己假设的最重要的发现,以及那些意外或显著的发现。文字和表格中的术语一定要一致。

每个表格和图都应该在正文中有明确提及,并按照顺序引用它们。

投稿的时候表格和图通常放在参考文献后面,每页只放一幅图或一张表。

表格的标题通常放在顶部,而图的标题通常放在底部。

一般杂志要求将表格或图作为单独的文件提交,而不是放在论文的Word文件中。注意,每个杂志对图的格式（例如 TIFF、JPEG 或 PNG）有不同的要求,不按要求提交文件会被退稿。

在正文中引用到图和表格的时候,注意以下规则:

• 除非必要,否则引用图形或表格的时候不应包括"see"。

• 引用的时候,用现在时,如:"Tables 2～3 and Figures 1 and 4～5 summarize…","Table 1 shows…"。

• 在括号中同时引用图和表时,用分号将它们分开,如"Table 2；Figure 1"。

• 多个图表的时候,用复数。连续的编码用连字符,否则用"and":"Figures 1～2","Tables 1 and 3","Figures 1～2；Tables 2 and 4"。

- 如果一个图包含多个图组（Panel），甚至亚组（Subpanel），用连字符分隔连续组或亚组，用逗号分隔非连续组，如："Figure 2B-C""Figure 3B,D"。

- 如果语法上有必要，则用"and"，不用连字符，如："There are endothelial cells and muscular cells(Figure 2B and C，respectively)"。因为有"respectively"，对应使用"and"，而不是用"Figure 2B-C"。或者这样描述："There are endothelial cells(Figure 2B) and muscular cells(Figure C)"。

- 引用图中或表格中的特定部分时尽可能避免使用所有格，如"Figure 2B inset"，"Figure 3 filled squares"，"Table 1 footnotes"。但有时候必须用所有格："Table 2's rightmost column"，"Table 2's 'Congenital anomalies'"。

参考文献

[1] Wang C，Schmid C H，Rones R，et al. A randomized trial of tai chi for fibromyalgia[J]. N Engl J Med，2010，363(8)：743 – 754.

[2] Fortier S M，Penke L R，Peters-Golden M. Illuminating the lung regenerative potential of prostanoids[J]. Sci Adv，2022，8(12)：eabp8322.

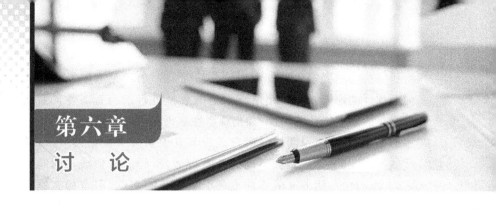

第六章
讨论

　　讨论是一篇文章很重要的部分，在结果已成定局的情况下，精彩的讨论可以给论文增色。讨论也是很多作者最不擅长写的部分。虽然讨论放在论文的最后，但研究过程中就可以加以准备：① 在收集到每一批数据的时候就要思考相应的讨论；② 在开展研究时不断收集相关的资料，这些都可能是很好的讨论素材。此外，可用预测读者、审稿人和编辑可能会提出的问题作为讨论的重点。

　　如果说前言的结构相当于漏斗，而讨论就相当于倒漏斗。因为讨论从具体的研究结果，即漏斗最狭窄的部分开始。总结部分一般用过去时态，回答前言中提出的研究问题或假说，包括对假设的肯定和否定。但关于对临床实践的影响的描述用现在时。倒漏斗的中间是具体的一系列针对研究结果的解析、不足之处、强项等的叙述。最后是倒漏斗最宽泛的部分，即对未来的展望。

第 1 节　讨论的组成

　　按照"CONSOTR"声明的建议，讨论应该包括以下三部分内容：① 局限性：研究的局限性，报告潜在偏倚和不精确的原因；② 可推广性：试验结果被推广的可能性（外部可靠性）；③ 解释：与结果相对应的机制解释，试验结果对未来医学的影响，未来医疗实践中采用新疗法的利弊，新疗法和其他疗法的对比。这些内容作者可以灵活整合。

　　这三部分内容通常可以通过以下段落展现：

　　第一段，应总结研究的结果，主要发现，和引言中提出的问题对应。对结果部分数据的引用应限于最重要的数字。

　　第二段，将论文从发现推进到解释。你的研究结果是否符合所研究疾病过程的生理学和病理学？提供一个理论来解释为什么事情会像你所预计的那样。不要超出结果中的数据进行没有针对性的解析。出现意外结果的原因也在此讨论，如出现阴性结果的可能原因。

第三段，应该说明你的研究是否与其他研究者或指南一致，并提出一致性或不一致的原因（例如不同的患者群体、不同的病情或不同的数据质量水平）。本段中引用的文献不应重复引言部分的文献（引言的文献只为研究提供了理论依据），而是应在您的研究、早期研究和同期进行的研究之间形成对比。不要过于详尽地描述他人研究的所有方面，而是关注那些与你自己的结论相关的内容。在引用其他研究时应避免使用作者名字。结果潜在偏倚和不精确的原因可以在此段体现。

第四段，清楚地阐明您的研究结果的临床意义。通过与文献对比来体现本研究的特点，本研究中每项数据的意义，对临床实践的影响。从你的研究作中可以学到哪些重要的知识？是否提高了患者生存率？是否有可能帮助诊断？

第五段，指出本研究的强项（Strengths of this study are…；Our study had several strengths）。把优势放在局限性之前。优势通常与设计有关：大样本、对照、双盲设计、更可靠的检测手段。如果你的设计比其他人的更严谨（例如，随机试验而不是观察性研究），这就是一个特别的优势。如果研究是多中心研究，那么此段可以指出可推广性很好（Strengths of this study are the large sample of adults and the use of multisource data to ascertain dementia）。

第六段，指出你的研究的局限性（There are limitations to this work；Our study also had some limitations.）。无论设计多么完善，没有一项研究是完美的。因此不用忌讳局限性，直截了当描述局限性，但不要过分批判。要在不影响研究有效性的前提下显示作者保持了深思熟虑和自我批评。这样，审稿人往往会支持你，减少他们的批评，更重要的是，它能让读者了解你的研究的实际局限性。对于一些研究来说，这些局限性是显而易见的：如样本量小，观察性研究，有混淆因素。承认研究的局限性是交流结果的重要组成部分。这表明你愿意提及和讨论你工作的弱点和不足之处。

有些研究确实很完善，但作者仍然需要写些不足之处。

不足之处的撰写要注意以下几点：

• 重点是研究设计和分析方法中的弱点，而不是结果。如果研究是单中心研究，那么可以认为可推广性方面是有局限的。报告潜在偏倚和不精确的地方可以在此段体现。

- 可以开门见山开始，然后进行必要的解释：

➢ This study has some limitations.

➢ This study has three main limitations. The first limitation is the small number of participants. However, also because the condition is rare, the findings of this study offer new, potentially useful information for this patient population.

➢ Our study has several limitations. We included only a small number of patients. However, our findings were clear and indicative. It is possible that the inclusion of more patients would have revealed further correlations in addition to those derived from the present analysis.

➢ Limitations of this study include its observational design and the low response rate(5.5%) of participants in UK Biobank, although studies have demonstrated this poor representativeness does not necessarily influence associations between physical activity and health outcomes. Reverse causation and residual confounding may still be presented. However, the large E-values showed this possibility is minimal.

➢ There are several limitations to the current trial. First, due to the coronavirus disease 2019(COVID-19) pandemic, the participant population is smaller than originally planned. However, given the power noted in this study, it is unlikely that population size was an impediment. Second, the population is relatively homogeneous and lacks racial and ethnic diversity, which should be addressed in future trials. Third, this report describes the findings of a short-term pre-specified primary outcome, 2 months after the last experimental session; long-term follow-up data from this controlled trial will be collected to assess durability of treatment. Last, given the subjective effects of MDMA, the blinding of participants was also challenging and possibly led to expectation effects. However, although blinding was not formally assessed during the study, when participants were contacted to be informed of their treatment assignment at the time of study unblinding it became apparent that at least 10% had inaccurately guessed their treatment arm. Although anecdotal, at least 7 of 44 participants in the placebo group (15.9%) inaccurately believed that they had received MDMA, and at least 2 of 46 participants in the MDMA group(4.3%) inaccurately believed that they had received placebo.

• 有些不是原则性的不足之处没有必要写。如在随访时候，随访日期没有严格按照计划，可能有几天的误差。

• 不要花费太多语言来解释为什么有局限性。

• 不要过分防御，避免以指责的方式指责其他人的研究。如果你的研究由于现实原因有特定的局限性，你可以指出这一点，但不要通过强调其他作者也有同样的不足之处来显示自己的不足之处的合理性。如："We had only 25 participants, but Smith et al. had only 12 and they still published their results."

最后一段应为总结段落，包括以下内容：① 本研究的主要发现和结论；强调你的发现的临床或基础科学意义；② 这些发现是否支持本研究提出的假设或目标；③ 基于这些发现是否可以提出新的理论和对未来进一步研究的建议或展望。如果没有合乎逻辑的下一步，就不要建议人们做进一步的研究。

第 2 节 RCT 的讨论

高质量随机对照临床研究在证据金字塔中占据最高位置。但 RCT 的实施往往不是一帆风顺。研究者都希望这样的结局：参与者很少退出、随访率高、研究没有提前终止、获得有临床意义和统计学差异的主要终点指标，获得明确的主要结果，以及合理一致的次要终点指标。当情况并非如此时，作者应该尽量在讨论中主动清楚地指出具有挑战性的问题，并进行合理的解析。

主要结果构成了讨论部分和文章结论的基础。临床试验还包括预先指定的二次分析、亚组分析、探索性结果和事后分析。对于主要结果之外的结果分析，必须指出错误推断的可能性，并明确这些结论是探索性的。

RCT 的解释往往很复杂，包括对整体研究设计中涉及的因素的理解、统计分析计划中的假设、观察到的事件率的解析、意外的结果的解析，以及研究结果的普遍性说明。此外，关于统计意义和临床重要性之间差异的描述、潜在利益和风险的平衡、干预的成本，以及特定患者和全部患者可能从干预中获得的价值。RCT 的解释必须考虑所有这些因素。

此外，可能还因为其他间接的因素而变得复杂，如试验提前停止（因无效或其他原因）、研究对象的依从性差、随访率低，或试验程序或预先指定的统计分析计划由于不可抗拒的原因（如新冠流行）需要修改。事后分析（Post hoc analysis）的目的也必须阐明。

下面是一些解析的案例。

对于事件发生率低于预期导致的阴性结果，可以这样解释：

➢ Among patients with AF, catheter ablation, compared with medical therapy, did not significantly reduce the primary composite end point. However, the estimated treatment effect of catheter ablation was affected by lower-than-expected event rates, which should be considered in interpreting the results of the trial.

➢ Among adults with hypertension, treating to a systolic blood pressure goal of less than 120 mmHg compared with a goal of less than 140 mmHg did not result in a significant reduction in the risk of probable dementia. Because of fewer than expected cases of dementia, the study may have been underpowered for this end point.

对于单中心的结果，需要强调验证性研究的重要性：

➢ However, these findings should be considered provisional until the generalizability is assessed in other institutions and settings.

对于一项试验，其结果差异可能符合预设的统计学显著性的标准，但观察到的效应没有达到临床有意义的差异，可以这样描写：

➢ Paracetamol plus ibuprofen significantly reduced morphine consumption compared with paracetamol alone. However, the combination did not result in a clinically important improvement over paracetamol alone, suggesting combination therapy may not be as effective as expected.

➢ Among patients with moderate to severe OA of the knee or hip and inadequate response to standard analgesics, tanezumab, compared with placebo, resulted in statistically significant improvements in pain scores, although the improvements were modest and tanezumab-treated patients had more joint safety events. Further research is needed to determine the clinical importance of these efficacy and adverse event findings.

对于主要结果不符合预设的显著性标准的试验，解释应强调观察到的效应大小：

➢ Although gastric bypass compared with sleeve gastrectomy was associated with greater percentage excess weight loss at 5 years, the difference was not statistically significant, based on the prespecified equivalence margins.

总之，对随机对照试验结果的解释必须结合问题的重要性、试验的设计和实施、可推广性、先前存在的证据和假设的一致性、统计检验和临床重要性来进行。

在报告临床试验(和其他类型的研究)结果时,使用"显著性(Significance)"一词和 P 值是一直处于争论中。一些人主张从临床试验结果的描述中删除"显著性"一词,只提供效应大小、95%的置信区间,作者使用其他方法来解释观察到的结果是否可能代表真实效应与抽样误差,以及效应大小是否重要。这些观点认为 $P=0.05$ 的阈值知识代表了一种历史传统,而不是一个合理的标准。

主张用统计学意义来描述临床试验的结果部分原因是监管机构(如美国 FDA)也是那么做的,而且有助于医生理解临床试验结果。通常,研究结果的统计学显著性差异(Statistically significant differences)或无统计学显著性差异(No statistically significant differences)和具有临床意义的效应大小"clinically important"是两个概念,要注意区别。

我们以论文"A randomized trial of tai chi for fibromyalgia"为例介绍临床研究的讨论描述[1]。

第一段是总结,包括有效性和安全性。

This randomized, controlled trial shows that tai chi is potentially a useful therapy for patients with fibromyalgia. The effect was evident in the FIQ score, a well-validated, multidimensional instrument for the assessment of fibromyalgia, and in other measures of pain and quality of life and was consistent with both subjective and objective assessments. The observed benefits exceeded the specified thresholds for clinically significant improvement in the FIQ score[30] and in the measures used to assess pain,[31] sleep quality,[24] depression,[32] and quality of life,[28,33] and these benefits were sustained at 24 weeks. No adverse events were reported in the study participants, indicating that tai chi is probably a safe therapy for patients with fibromyalgia.

这项随机对照试验表明,太极拳对纤维肌痛患者可能是一种有效的治疗方法。这种作用在 FIQ 评分中很明显,FIQ 评分是一种经过充分验证的多维度评估纤维肌痛的工具,在其他疼痛和生活质量指标中也很明显,并且与主观和客观评估一致。研究中观察到的益处超过了 FIQ 评分[30]和用于评估疼痛[31]、睡眠质量[24]、抑郁[32]、和生活质量的指标[28,33]的临床显著改善的规定阈值,这些益处在 24 周时仍然保持。研究参与者中没有不良事件报告,这表明太极可能是纤维肌痛患者的安全疗法。

此段前面用现在时(shows),因为作者认为,结合以往的研究,这个结论是可靠的。但在提出此次研究的证据的时候,用的过去时(The effect was evident in …)。此外,作者指出这些指标的改善程度超过了行业公认的有临床价值的最小值。这里要用参考文献指出这些最小值的出处。这也是我们强调的要在文献背景下证明本研究的价值,不能王婆卖瓜自卖自夸。

第二段通过文献对比支持本研究的结论是可靠的。

Our results are consistent with those of a previous, nonrandomized trial of tai chi for fibromyalgia, as well as with the findings in other studies showing the benefits of tai chi with regard to musculoskeletal pain, depression, and quality of life[13,34]. Our findings are also consistent with observations from other clinical trials and meta-analyses that support the benefits of physical exercise and mind-body practice for symptom management in fibromyalgia[35-41].

我们的结果与之前一项太极治疗纤维肌痛的非随机试验的结果一致,也与其他研究的结果一致[13,34],我们的发现也与其他临床试验和荟萃分析的观察结果一致,这些观察结果支持体育锻炼和身心练习对纤维肌痛症状管理的益处[35-41]。

注意,"are consistent with"和"are also consistent with"用现在时。

第三段对结果进行解释。临床研究一般不做机制研究,因为相应的机制研究一般都在先前的细胞和动物上完成后才能转化到临床。因此,对疗效的解释主要是引用文献中的临床前研究数据,也包括早期的探索性临床研究和类似的临床研究。如:

The biologic mechanisms by which tai chi might affect the clinical course of fibromyalgia remain unknown. As a complex, multicomponent intervention, tai chi may act through many intermediate variables along the pathway to improved health outcomes. Physical exercise has been shown to increase muscle strength and blood lactate levels in some patients with fibromyalgia[42]. Mind-body interventions may improve psychosocial well-being, increase confidence, and help patients overcome fear of pain. 43 Furthermore, controlled breathing and movements promote a restful state and mental tranquility, which may raise pain thresholds and help break the "pain cycle"[44]. All these components may influence neuroendocrine and immune function as well as neurochemical and analgesic pathways that lead to enhanced physical, psychological, and psychosocial well-being and overall quality of life in patients with fibromyalgia[40,45,46].

太极拳如何影响纤维肌痛临床过程的生物学机制尚不清楚。作为一种复杂的多因素干预，太极拳可能通过许多中间变量来改善健康结果。体育锻炼已被证明可以增加一些纤维肌痛患者的肌肉力量和血乳酸水平[42]。身心干预可以改善心理健康，增加信心，帮助患者克服疼痛恐惧[43]。此外，控制呼吸和运动可以促进休息状态和精神安宁，这可能会提高疼痛阈值，帮助打破"疼痛循环"[44]。所有这些成分都可能影响神经内分泌和免疫功能以及神经化学和镇痛途径，从而增强纤维肌痛患者的身体、心理和社会心理健康以及整体生活质量[40,45,46]。

第四段是指出研究的不足之处。写不足之处的时候通常要解析相应的原因，并指出这些不足之处不会影响结果的正确性。

Our study had some limitations. We did not use a double-blind study design, since this would have required the use of sham tai chi, for which no validated approach currently exists. Devising a sham mind-body intervention poses a set of unique challenges when one attempts to separate the various mind and body components. Nevertheless, the development of some forms of sham intervention for use in future studies of tai chi is a desirable goal. To minimize the influence of preexisting beliefs and expectations with respect to tai chi (e.g., its possible placebo effect), we informed participants only that the study was designed to test the effects of two different types of exercise training programs, one of which was combined with education. De-emphasizing tai chi may have lessened participants' expectations and minimized biases. Notably, the baseline outcome expectations of benefit from an exercise intervention were similar in the tai chi and control groups (3.7±0.8 and 3.9±0.7, respectively), indicating that our neutral presentation of the interventions may have been successful.

我们的研究有一些局限性。我们没有采用双盲研究设计，因为这需要使用模拟太极，目前还没有有效的方法做到。当研究者试图分离干预的不同心理和身体作用因素时，设计一个虚假的心理-身体干预是很难的。然而，开发某种形式的模拟太极拳用于未来的太极拳研究是一个理想的目标。为了尽量减少对太极拳的现有信念和期望的影响（例如，其可能的安慰剂效应），我们仅告知参与者，该研究旨在测试两种不同类型的运动训练的效果，其中一种与教育相结合。淡化太极拳可能降低了参与者的期望，并将偏离降至最低。值得注意的是，太极组和对照组对运动干预获益的基线结果预期相似

（分别为 3.7 ± 0.8 和 3.9 ± 0.7），这表明我们对干预的中性描述应该是成功的。

第一句"*Our study had some limitations.*"可以用现在时，也可以用过去时。

The fact that treatment was delivered by a single tai chi master at a single center also potentially limits the generalizability of our results. However, the group of patients with poor health status at baseline may in general resemble patients with fibromyalgia. For these reasons, it would be prudent to further explore the benefits of tai chi for fibromyalgia in other settings with other instructors. Since tai chi is a complex mind-body intervention with a variety of active ingredients, such as social support, relaxation, and cognitive behavioral elements[47], assessment of its placebo effect might require separate evaluations of these ingredients. Finally, we followed participants for only 24 weeks, so the long-term effectiveness of tai chi in patients with fibromyalgia remains to be determined.

治疗是由一位太极拳师傅在一个中心进行的，这也可能限制了我们结果的可推广性。然而，基线时健康状况不佳的患者组通常代表了纤维肌痛患者。出于这些原因，需要进一步证明其他师傅其他场合下太极拳对纤维肌痛的益处。由于太极拳是一种复杂的身心干预，含有多种有益成分，如社会支持、放松和认知行为元素[47]，评估其安慰剂效应可能需要对这些成分进行单独评估。最后，我们只跟踪了24周，因此太极拳对纤维肌痛患者的长期疗效仍有待确定。

这一段在讨论研究的不足之处时讨论了研究结果的可普及性较差。此外，没有对安慰剂效应进行评估也是不足之处。

最后一段是总结：

In conclusion, our preliminary findings indicate that tai chi may be a useful treatment in the multidisciplinary management of fibromyalgia. Longer-term studies involving larger clinical samples are warranted to assess the generalizability of our findings and to deepen our understanding of this promising therapeutic approach.

总之，我们的初步发现表明，太极拳可能是多学科治疗纤维肌痛的有效方法。具有更大临床样本的长期研究有助于评估我们发现的可推广性，并加深我们对这种有前途的治疗方法的理解。

最后一段关于研究的总结部分一般用过去时，展望或结论部分则用现在时。但如果作者认为该研究的结论非常可靠，可作为定论，可采用现在时。

每项研究都有其局限性,一定要指出并说明。不要对不好的结果避而不谈,审稿专家会看到的。避而不谈只会让审稿人认为研究者居然不知道设计中的瑕疵。诚实会使论文更有说服力。

但不好的结果(或阴性结果)不属于不足之处的范围。

同样,好的研究在设计的时候可能有"过人之处";结果又有可能有重要发现,因此要明确指出本研究的强项和优点。为了强调本研究的重要性,有时候难免要对他人的相关研究的局限性(缺点)进行分析。分析他人的研究要尊重对方和客观,比如尽量强调你的数据对他人证据的补充(什么是已知的?什么是新的?两者有何关联?)。通过与其他研究进行比较明确指出本研究"重要性"或相似之处,以及可能的原因。如下面的讨论,作者指出,作为肾移植的诱导疗法 MSC 有可能比传统的 IL-2 抗体更好,因为病人的肾功能恢复更快[2]:

We found that autologous MSC recipients had faster renal function recovery during the first month, displayed fewer adverse events and had reduced opportunistic infections than controls. Thus, autologous MSCs may replace anti-IL-2 receptor antibodies and may allow for using lower CNIs maintenance doses without compromising patient safety and graft outcome.

参考文献

[1] Wang C, Schmid C H, Rones R, et al. A randomized trial of tai chi for fibromyalgia[J]. N Engl J Med, 2010,363(8):743 - 754.

[2] Tan J, Wu W, Xu X, et al. Induction therapy with autologous mesenchymal stem cells in living-related kidney transplants: a randomized controlled trial [J]. JAMA,2012,307(11):1169 - 1177.

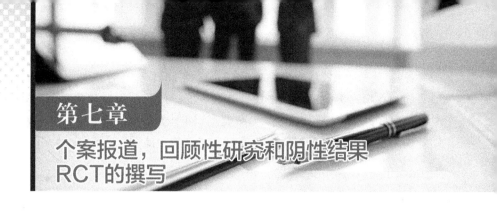

第七章
个案报道，回顾性研究和阴性结果RCT的撰写

第1节　个案报道

　　个案报道(或病例报告，Case report)，也称为病例研究(Case study)，是对患者临床过程的详细描述。报道的病例必须足够独特、罕见或有趣，以便其他医疗专业人员可以从中学到新的知识(包括作者的见解)。值得报道或杂志/读者感兴趣的个案报告包括首次发现的罕见病、不寻常的疾病表现、多种疾病首次同时出现、新的诊断方法、新的治疗方法，以及特殊解剖变异等。

　　病例报道在医学界是一个历史悠久的传统。从希波克拉底(公元前460年—公元前370年)，甚至可以说从古埃及医学的莎草纸记录(公元前1600年)到现代，很多医生描述了很多有趣的病例。在我国传统医学中，写医案也是习以为常的。事实上，很多现在医学知识的常识，最早都是以个案报道的形式出现的，如卡波西肉瘤[1]。早期的病例报道只不过是同事之间关于各自医疗实践中看到的独特而有趣的病人的个人交流。这种轶事报道已经发展成为一种公认的学术出版形式，采用标题、摘要、介绍(背景)、病例介绍(Case presentation)、讨论、结论和参考文献等的格式。许多医学期刊发表病例报道，包括《NEJM》和《Lancet》。有些专业有专门的个案报道杂志。

　　个案报道通常讨论单个患者的情况，不是有目的的研究，原则上不需要伦理批准，而且如果不暴露患者信息的话，也不需要获得患者的知情同意。也有些杂志要求知情同意。如果包括一个以上的病人，这种病例系列报道一般认为属于研究，需要获得伦理委员会批准和患者的知情同意。

　　病例报道的撰写建议参考"CARE(CAse REport)指南"(表

7.1)[2]。CARE 指南是 2012 年 10 月由 18 个与会者在美国密西根大学制定的。在撰写之前可尝试查找以前发表的类似病例报道作为示例。在 PubMed 上以疾病为主题，在左侧"文章类型"(article type)菜单选择"Case reports"。如果在菜单没有看到这个选项，点击"附加过滤器"(additional filters)增加。

表 7.1　CARE 项目清单

标题	项目	项目描述
题目	1	标题中含有"个案报道"(case report)，方便读者检索
关键词	2	概括该病的 2～5 个关键词。关键词有助于读者查找到该个案报道
摘要	3a	该报道的特点是什么？它能给医学文献增添什么（为什么要写该个案报道）？
	3b	患者的主要症状和重要的临床结果
	3c	主要诊断，治疗干预措施和产生的效果
	3d	从该报道中能得到什么经验
前言	4	用 1～2 段概述该个案报道的背景和来龙去脉，为什么该病例是独一无二的，并附上参考文献
患者信息	5a	事先确定患者的人口统计信息及其他患者的特殊信息（如年龄、性别、种族和职业相关的资料）
	5b	患者的主要病症
	5c	包括遗传信息在内的医学、家庭及社会心理史（也可以看时间轴）
	5d	相关的以往干预措施和结果
临床结果	6	描述相关的体检和其他有意义的临床结果
时间轴	7	来自患者以往病史的重要信息
诊断评估	8a	诊断方法（如体检、实验室检查、影像学检查）
	8b	诊断面临的挑战（如设备、经济和文化）
	8c	诊断推理
	8d	预后特征（如肿瘤的分级）
治疗的干预措施	9a	干预的类型（如药物、外科手术、自我调理）
	9b	干预措施的实施（如剂量、强度和持续时间）
	9c	干预措施的改变（阐述原因）
随访和结果	10a	医生和患者评估结果

标题	项目	项目描述
	10b	重要的随访诊断方法和检测结果
	10c	干预措施的持续和耐受性(评估方法)
	10d	不良反应和意外事件
讨论	11a	讨论该病例中所用方法的有效性和局限性。该病例报告的亮点和不足之处
	11b	讨论相关的文献
	11c	结果的推论原理(如可能的因果关系和普遍性)
	11d	病例有用的经验和信息
患者的观点	12	必要时患者分享他们对所接受治疗方法的看法
知情同意	13	患者是否有签署知情同意书？如果要求的话,请提供

　　个案报道一般比较简短,但有些个案比较复杂,篇幅也会很长。在下面的例子中,我们分别介绍了一短一长两个例子。

　　我们先介绍短的例子,题目是"Successful osimertinib rechallenge after relapse following adjuvant osimertinib：a case report"[3]。题目明确说明是个案。在 Introduction 部分,作者写道：

　　Adjuvant osimertinib in resectable EGFR-mutated lung cancer resulted in significantly increased disease free[1] and overall survival[2] in the ADAURA trial（NCT02511106）. For patients who relapse after completion of 3 years of adjuvant osimertinib，it is unclear whether rechallenge of osimertinib would be efficacious or whether unfavorable mechanisms of resistance may arise at relapse after an osimertinib-free interval. This uncertainty is reflected in heterogeneous subsequent treatment in the ADAURA study，in which 41％ of patients received osimertinib，38％ received another EGFR inhibitor，25％ received platinum-based chemotherapy，and small numbers received other therapies.[2] Outcomes data for these subsequent treatments are not available，reflecting an unmet need. Here，we describe complete response（CR）to osimertinib rechallenge in two patients who participated in the ADUARA study and relapsed after 3 years of adjuvant osimertinib.

　　在 ADAURA 试验（NCT02511106）中,奥希替尼辅助治疗可切除的 EGFR 突变肺癌可显著提高无病生存期[1] 和总生存期[2]。对于奥希替尼辅助治疗 3 年后复发的患者,尚不清楚再次使用奥希替尼是否有效,或者在未服用奥希替尼的间隔期后复发的肿瘤是否会出现耐药。这种不确定性反映在 ADAURA 研究的异质性后续治疗中,其中 41％的患者接受了奥西替尼,38％接受了其他 EGFR 抑制剂,25％接受了铂类化疗,少数接受了其他治疗[2]。目前还没有这些后续治疗的结果数据,因此这些患者有未被满足的需求。在这里,我们介绍了两名参加 ADUARA 研究的患者在 3 年的奥西替尼辅助治疗后复发,再次服用奥西替尼后完全缓解(CR)。

在背景介绍中作者明确指出,奥西替尼辅助治疗后肺癌复发是否可以再用奥西替尼治疗从来没有人报道过,这是本文的一个新颖性。其次,理论上再用奥西替尼可能无效,但结果两个患者都有效,这个意外的发现是第二个新颖性。

此段中第一句 resulted 用过去式,代表过去的研究。"This uncertainty is …"用了现在时,代表了一个现在的推论,后面的"received"用过去式。最后的"Here, we describe …"是个案报道的常用句式,用现在时,但后面的"participated"和"relapsed"用过去时。

注意,"disease free survival"和"overall survival"后面不要加"time"。"osimertinib-free"指停用"osimertinib"。

接下去是"Case Report"部分。第一段描述了首个患者的治疗史。第一句的年龄描述用现在时,表明撰写文章时的患者年龄,其他用过去时。"unremarkable"是体检的常用语,指结果正常,或未发现异常:

Patient 1 is a 59-year-old female nonsmoker who underwent right lower lobectomy for stage IIA lung adenocarcinoma with EGFR L858R mutation, followed by 3 years of adjuvant osimertinib without adjuvant chemotherapy. With osimertinib, the patient suffered low-grade cutaneous toxicity, mucositis, and neutropenia. Six months after completion of treatment, routine surveillance computed tomography of the chest, abdomen, and pelvis detected a new 9-mm nodule in the posterior right lower lobe of the lung with surrounding ground-glass changes (Fig. 1A), and multiple prominent mediastinal lymph nodes. The patient was asymptomatic with an unremarkable physical examination.

患者 1 是一名 59 岁的非吸烟女性,因 EGFR L858R 突变的 IIA 期肺腺癌接受了右下肺叶切除术,随后接受了 3 年的奥希替尼辅助治疗,没有辅助化疗。奥西替尼治疗期间患者出现低度皮肤毒性、黏膜炎和中性粒细胞减少症。治疗完成 6 个月后,胸部、腹部和骨盆的常规 CT 随访发现肺右下叶后侧有一个新发的 9mm 结节,周围有磨玻璃样改变(图 1A),并有多个明显的纵隔淋巴结。病人无症状,体格检查正常。

第二段是基因检测结果和再次治疗的结果。再次开始治疗用了"recommenced",是比较正式的书面语。

Mediastinal lymph node biopsy confirmed recurrent lung adenocarcinoma exhibiting EGFR L858R mutation and TP53 mutation without other EGFR alteration such as C797S mutation or copy number variation in ERBB2 and MET. The patient recommenced osimertinib, achieving a CR to therapy, with resolution of the previously exhibited pulmonary nodule and no lymphadenopathy on restaging computed tomography after 2 months of treatment (Fig. 1B).

纵隔淋巴结活检证实性肺腺癌复发,表现为 EGFR L858R 突变和 TP53 突变,无其他 EGFR 改变,如 C797S 突变或 ERBB2 和 MET 拷贝数变化。患者重新使用奥西替尼,治疗 2 个月后 CT 再检查显示先前的肺结节消失,没有淋巴结病变治疗,达到 CR(图 1B)。

第三段描述服药后期的临床进展:

The duration of the response was 14.8 months. The patient remained clinically well with low-volume disease and continued osimertinib beyond radiographic progression until clinical progression after 32 months. She commenced second-line carboplatin and pemetrexed with radiologic partial response.

反应持续时间为 14.8 个月。患者临床表现良好,病灶体积小,并继续使用奥西替尼,即使有影像学进展也未停药,直到 32 个月后出现临床进展才停药。她开始使用二线卡铂和培美曲塞,放射学检测显示部分反应。

第二个患者的描述大致和第一个患者一样。这里"commence"和"start","begin"的意思一样,可以互换,但更加正式:

Patient 2 is an 80-year-old female nonsmoker who underwent right middle lobectomy for stage IIA lung adenocarcinoma with EGFR exon 21 mutation, followed by four cycles of adjuvant cisplatin and vinorelbine and 3 years of adjuvant osimertinib. With osimertinib, the patient suffered mild gastrointestinal toxicity. Twenty-six months after completion of osimertinib, her disease recurred in the brain and lungs (Fig. 2A). Biopsy was not performed as the recurrence was small volume.

患者 2 是一名 80 岁的女性非吸烟者,因 EGFR 外显子 21 突变的ⅡA 期肺腺癌接受了右中肺叶切除术,随后接受了 4 个周期的顺铂和维诺瑞滨辅助治疗和 3 年的奥希替尼辅助治疗。服用奥西替尼期间患者出现轻度胃肠道毒性。奥西替尼治疗结束 26 个月后出现脑部和肺部复发(图 2A)。复发的肿瘤体积小,因此未行活检。

After cranial radiotherapy, she commenced first-line osimertinib for recurrent disease, achieving radiologic CR after 9 months, which is currently ongoing at 14 months after commencing treatment (Fig. 2B).

脑部放疗后患者开始一线奥西替尼治疗复发性疾病,9 个月后达到放射学 CR,目前处于开始治疗后的第 14 个月(图 2B)。

接下去是"Discussion"部分。讨论的第一段介绍了一些新的背景知识,和"Introduction"相呼应:

Acquired resistance to osimertinib in the metastatic setting is inevitable. Mechanisms of resistance in the metastatic setting are heterogeneous and differ between first-line and second-line metastatic treatment[3]. Whether recurrent tumors after adjuvant therapy will

be populated by resistant clones, and whether osimertinib rechallenge will, therefore, become futile, is unknown in the absence of basic science or observational data. Indeed, anticipating acquired resistance in this setting, some authors have proposed the investigation of alternative treatment sequencing in which first generation EGFR tyrosine kinase inhibitors are used in the adjuvant setting, with osimertinib reserved for subsequent treatment on relapse[4].

转移性肿瘤对奥希替尼的获得性耐药是不可避免的。转移性肿瘤的耐药机制是多样的,一线和二线转移性治疗的耐药机制也不同[3]。辅助治疗后复发的肿瘤是否由耐药克隆性肿瘤细胞组成,以及奥西替尼的再次使用是否会因此变得无效,都是未知的,没有基础科学或观察数据。事实上,因为预计在这种情况下肿瘤会获得性耐药,一些作者提出了其他的治疗策略,其中第一代 EGFR 酪氨酸激酶抑制剂先用于辅助治疗,奥希替尼保留用于复发后的后续治疗[4]。

讨论的第二段是结果和相应的解析(通常结果放在第一段,第二段进行解析):

It is interesting that our reported cases revealed durable responses with rechallenge of osimertinib regardless of relapse-free interval after cessation of adjuvant osimertinib (6 and 26 mo). This observation and the results of the serial molecular panel in patient 1 suggest an absence of acquired resistance mechanisms at the time of relapse，therefore，maintaining sensitivity to osimertinib.

有趣的是,我们报道的病例显示,无论停止辅助奥希替尼后的无复发间隔多长（6 个月和 26 个月）,再次服用奥希替尼的患者都有持久的反应。这一观察结果和患者 1 的系列分子研究结果表明复发时没有出现获得性耐药,因此肿瘤对奥希替尼仍然敏感。

讨论的第三段描述了这个案例的价值和不足之处:

Our case series provides some observational data supporting the role of osimertinib as the first-line subsequent treatment on relapse after completion of adjuvant treatment. Limitations of our study include the lack of serial biopsy and molecular panel in patient 2 and the small patient numbers. These limitations raise the unanswered question of whether a proportion of patients who relapse after completion of adjuvant osimertinib may harbor resistance mechanisms that would render osimertinib rechallenge ineffective.

我们的病例系列提供了一些观察性数据,支持奥希替尼继续作为奥希替尼辅助治疗完成后复发的一线后续治疗。本研究的局限性包括第二个患者没有做连续活检和分子检测,此外患者人数少。这些局限性提出了一个悬而未决的问题,即是否有一部分患者在完成奥希替尼辅助治疗后复发的时候可能产生了对奥希替尼的耐药,导致再次服用无效。

最后是"Conclusion"部分。第一句的结论用的是过去式,仅代表此两位患者的结果。"Future prospective studies are warranted to confirm …"是常用的句式:

Osimertinib rechallenge was an effective subsequent treatment in our reported cases. We believe that future prospective studies are warranted to confirm the best treatment approach in this population and to define the genomic landscape of such tumors.

在我们报道的病例中,奥西替尼再次治疗是一种有效的后续治疗。我们相信,未来有必要在这一人群中开展前瞻性研究,确认最佳治疗方法,并确定此类肿瘤的基因图谱。

接下来我们介绍第二个较长的范文,题目是"Polysubstance-induced relapse of schizoaffective disorder refractory to high-dose antipsychotic medications：a case report"[4]。标题明确显示是个案。该范文的每一个部分都较长,各部分的比例适当。作者报道了一例毒品诱发的分裂情感性障碍复发患者,这个病例的特征是高剂量抗精神病药物治疗无效。背景介绍的第一段作者对严重精神疾病患者使用毒品的情况做了介绍。这是一个大的背景,相当于漏斗的顶部,引用了 4 个参考文献

Illicit drug use is a significant problem among persons with major mental illness. The 2010 Australian National Survey of Psychotic Disorders <u>reported</u> psychoactive substance abuse in 63% of men and 41% of women with psychosis, compared with 12% of men and 6% of women in the general population[1]. This high comorbidity represents one of the biggest barriers to effective management of schizophrenia and related disorders since substance use can reduce compliance with medications, exacerbate psychosis, precipitate a major relapse of illness requiring hospitalization, and increase treatment resistance over the lifetime of the illness[2,3]. <u>It has been hypothesized</u> that the high comorbidity of illicit drug use and chronic psychotic disorders may reflect an inherent neurobiological vulnerability to developing a substance abuse disorder, a strategy to alleviate symptoms of the primary mental illness or the adverse effects of medications, or that patterns of use may simply reflect the local availability of illicit substances[4].

非法药物使用是一个严重问题。2010 年澳大利亚全国精神病调查报告称,63% 的男性和 41% 的女性精神病患者滥用精神活性物质,而在普通人群中,这一比例为男性 12% 和女性 6%[1]。这种高的共病发生率是有效管理精神分裂症和相关疾病的最大障碍之一,因为毒品使用会降低治疗药物的依从性,加剧精神病,促使疾病复发,需要住院治疗,并增加患者一生中的治疗耐药性[2,3]。据推测,毒品使用和慢性精神障碍的共病高发生率可能反映了一种固有的神经生物学脆弱性,即容易发生药物滥用,当地毒品的可及性可能和原发性精神疾病症状或药物不良反应,或者使用模式有关[4]。

这段中,"reported"用过去式,其他描述用现在时。" It has been hypothesized"用现在完成时。我们前面介绍过现在完成时可以表达特殊的意境,如过去开始、正在进行的行动,暗示过去的行动对现在有影响。

背景介绍的第二段作者对毒品做了介绍,并过渡到具体的兴奋剂和冰毒。这是一个更加具体的背景,相当于漏斗的中部。引用了 4 个参考文献:

The illicit drugs of choice for persons with major psychotic disorders are most frequently cannabis followed by stimulants such as cocaine, amphetamine, and methamphetamine. Approximately 11% of persons

with schizophrenia abuse cannabis and stimulants concurrently[2]. One psychostimulant of particular interest is crystalline methamphetamine, also known as "ice", which is both highly addictive and growing in popularity. Ice use reportedly more than doubled from 22% to 50% among illicit amphetamine users in Australia between 2010 and 2013[5]. The frequency of daily or weekly ice use also doubled from 12.4% to 25% over the same period[5]. Correspondingly there have been increased public concerns about the drug's detrimental impact on mental and physical health, social functioning, crime rates, and public safety since intoxicated users have a propensity towards hostility and interpersonal violence[6]. Escalation in the use of ice has thus resulted in a predictable rise in methamphetamine-related presentations to Australian emergency departments[6,7].

患有严重精神障碍的人最常选择的非法药物是大麻,其次是兴奋剂,如可卡因、安非他明和甲基苯丙胺。大约11%的精神分裂症患者同时滥用大麻和兴奋剂[2]。一种特别令人关注的精神兴奋剂是结晶甲基苯丙胺,也被称为冰毒,它容易上瘾,而且越来越普遍。据报道,2010年至2013年间,澳大利亚非法安非他明使用者中冰毒的使用率从22%增加到50%,翻了一倍多[5]。在同一时期,每天或每周使用冰毒的频率也从12.4%增加到25%[5]。相应地,由于吸毒后有敌意和人际暴力倾向,公众对毒品对身心健康、社会功能、犯罪率和公共安全的有害影响的担忧也越来越多[6]。因此可以预见冰毒使用的增加会导致澳大利亚急诊科接诊的与甲基苯丙胺有关的患者增加[6,7]。

背景介绍的最后一段作者对甲基苯丙胺滥用导致的急性精神病复发做了介绍。这是一个和本病例直接相关的具体背景,相当于漏斗的尖部。引用了6篇参考文献:

A relatively common illness associated with habitual or binge use of methamphetamine is a transient psychotic reaction. For individuals without a history of primary psychotic illness, this psychotic reaction is referred to as methamphetamine-induced acute psychosis. Comparatively, for individuals with a pre-existing primary psychotic disorder, this psychotic reaction is referred to as an acute psychotic relapse precipitated by methamphetamine abuse. The clinical features of methamphetamine-induced acute psychosis commonly include hallucinatory experiences and persecutory delusions accompanied by hostile behavior[8]. Bizarre delusions, formal thought disorder, or negative symptoms are less common[8-10].

Consequently, methamphetamine-induced acute psychosis can appear remarkably similar to acute paranoid schizophrenia[11]. The time course of methamphetamine-induced acute psychosis is normally brief, lasting hours to a few days, with patients usually making a full recovery with abstinence[12]. It has been reported that patients with methamphetamine-induced acute psychosis normally respond well to antipsychotic medications[13]. However, there have been very few reports of severely unwell patients with either methamphetamine-induced acute psychosis or methamphetamine-precipitated psychotic relapse who respond poorly to antipsychotic medications and the safety issues that arise in this scenario.

与经常性或大剂量甲基苯丙胺有关的一种相对常见的疾病是短暂的精神反应。对于没有原发性精神病病史的个体，这种精神病反应被称为甲基苯丙胺诱发的急性精神病。相比之下，对于先前存在原发性精神病的个体，这种精神病反应被称为甲基苯丙胺滥用导致的急性精神病复发。甲基苯丙胺诱发的急性精神病的临床特征通常包括幻觉和迫害妄想，并伴有敌对行为[8]。奇怪的妄觉、思维障碍或阴性症状不太常见[8-10]。因此，甲基苯丙胺诱发的急性精神病与急性偏执型精神分裂症非常相似[11]。甲基苯丙胺引起的急性精神病病程通常很短，持续数小时至数天，患者通常在戒断后完全康复[12]。据报道，甲基苯丙胺诱发的急性精神病通常对抗精神病药物反应良好[13]。然而，关于甲基苯丙胺诱发的重症急性精神病或甲基苯丙胺诱发的重症精神病复发的报道很少，这些患者对抗精神病药物反应不佳，导致安全性问题。

这段用现在时描述基本常识。" It has been reported"和"However, there have been very few reports"用现在完成时，暗示本案例和这些报道有关。

接下去是具体的患者描述（Case presentation），用的是过去式。首先是患者的人口统计信息，主要病症和以往的干预措施等：

A 30-year-old white man was brought to our emergency department by the police under the Mental Health Act in an aggressive and combative state threatening suicide and homicide. His presentation was precipitated by daily cannabis use and multiple binges of ice over the prior month. His past psychiatric history included childhood attention deficit hyperactivity disorder (ADHD) and schizoaffective disorder which was managed on a Community Treatment Order with fortnightly 300 mg zuclopenthixol decanoate intramuscular injections. His past medical history was remarkable for polysubstance abuse. From 15 years of age he regularly used tobacco, alcohol, and cannabis, and sporadically used heroin, hallucinogens, ecstasy, and amphetamines. In terms of family history, his father had ADHD and one historical episode of manic psychotic illness requiring treatment with medication and electroconvulsive therapy. His male sibling was deceased from suicide after protracted illness with major depression and binge eating disorder. Our patient had a long history of transient living and difficulty sustaining regular employment in bricklaying. At the time of presentation, he was living in a shared residence and using ice most days in the context of interpersonal conflict, unemployment, financial stressors, and housing stressors.

警方根据《精神卫生法》将一名 30 岁的白人男子带到我们的急诊室,他表现出咄咄逼人、好斗的状态,扬言要自杀和杀人。他的症状是由于前一个月每天吸食大麻和多次吸食冰毒导致的。他过去的精神病史包括儿童注意缺陷多动障碍(ADHD)和分裂情感性障碍,根据社区治疗法规每两周肌注 300 mg 珠氯噻醇。他有滥用多种药物的病史。从 15 岁起,他就经常吸烟、喝酒、吸大麻,偶尔吸食海洛因、致幻剂、摇头丸和安非他明。在家族史方面,他的父亲患有多动症并有一段躁狂精神病病史,需要药物治疗和电休克治疗。他的兄弟在长期患有严重抑郁症和暴食症后自杀。病人有很长一段居无定所的生活史,并且很难维持正常的瓦工工作。在出现症状时,他住在一个共享的住所,在人际冲突、失业、经济压力和住房压力的背景下,他大部分日子都在使用冰毒。

接下来的一段包括了相关的体检和其他有意义的临床结果:

On his arrival at our emergency department, six-point mechanical restraint was required for his safety and for the safety of the staff and co-patients. An initial physical examination revealed Glasgow Coma Score of 14 …tachycardic pulse 110 beats/minute, blood pressure 125/63 mmHg, fingertip oxygen saturation 95% on room air, and tympanic temperature 36.1℃. A subsequent physical examination revealed that his pupils were equal … He claimed that he had been stabbed in the torso by his flatmate despite no evidence of any external injuries. A full blood examination, C-reactive protein test, random blood glucose test, liver function tests, thyroid function tests, and ethanol level were unremarkable … His dehydration was treated with 1 L of 0.9% normal saline solution administered intravenously due to his refusal to take food and fluids orally.

当他到我们的急诊科时,为了他的安全,以及工作人员和其他病人的安全,我们要求对他进行六点式机械约束。初步体检显示格拉斯哥昏迷评分为14分……心动过速110次/分,血压125/63 mmHg,室内空气指尖氧饱和度95%,鼓室温度36.1℃。随后的体格检查显示他的瞳孔大小相等……他声称自己被他的室友刺伤了躯干,尽管没有任何外伤的证据。全血检查、C反应蛋白测试、随机血糖测试、肝功能测试、甲状腺功能测试和乙醇水平无明显异常……由于他拒绝口服食物和液体,静脉注射1 L 0.9%生理盐水以治疗脱水。

接下来的3段包括了诊断方法、干预的药物和随访结果:

Rapid sedation was commenced with ziprasidone, lorazepam, droperidol, and zuclopenthixol acetate (Table 1). Benztropine was administered for prophylaxis against extrapyramidal side effects of the antipsychotic medications. The level of sedation attained was unsatisfactory as he remained severely agitated and combative interspersed with only brief periods of drowsiness …

开始使用齐拉西酮、劳拉西泮、哌啶醇和醋酸珠氯噻醇快速镇静(表1)。苯托品用于预防抗精神病药物的锥体外系副作用。镇静的效果并不令人满意,因为他仍然非常激动和好斗,只是偶尔有短暂的困倦……

After psychiatric review in our emergency department he was transferred to a closed seclusion room on the psychiatric ward. He scored maximally on the Dynamic Appraisal of Situational Aggression (DASA) scale[14]. Droperidol 25 mg and lorazepam 2 mg were administered intramuscularly four times a day under physical restraint. His vital signs were measured every 4 hours; they remained within normal limits and no extrapyramidal side effects were observed.

在我们的急诊科进行精神检查后,他被转移到精神科病房的一个封闭的隔离室。他在情景攻击动态评价(DASA)量表上得分最高[14]。在身体约束下肌注氟哌啶醇25 mg,劳拉西泮2 mg,每日4次。每4小时测量一次生命体征;它们保持在正常范围内,未观察到锥体外系副作用。

A psychiatric review was re-attempted 27 hours into closed seclusion … This behavior continued despite treatment which consisted of high-dose antipsychotic medications and lorazepam for 3 days. … there was a sudden improvement in his mental state at 96 hours of treatment … A repeat urine drug screen revealed a trace amount of methamphetamine.

在隔离27小时后再次进行了精神病学检查……尽管服用了大剂量抗精神病药物和劳拉西泮3天,这种行为仍在继续……在96小时的治疗后,他的精神状态突然好转……再次尿检结果显示有微量甲基苯丙胺。

He was engaged and cooperative for the first time at review 120-hours post-presentation … There were no signs of major mental illness that required ongoing in-patient treatment, and he was discharged home on a Community Treatment Order with continued zuclopenthixol decanoate depot medication. After discharge, he engaged regularly with our mental health service to receive his depot … He had no further admissions to acute psychiatric units during a period of 18 months post-discharge.

在入院后 120 小时的检查中他第一次能够安静配合……没有任何需要持续住院治疗的重大精神疾病的迹象，根据社区治疗规定，他出院回家，继续服用珠氯噻醇。出院后，他定期到我们的心理健康服务处接受治疗……在出院后的 18 个月内，他没有再来过急诊精神科。

讨论的第一段，作者对和本病例相关的文献进行了复习（略）。一般来说，第一段可以对本病例做个总结。

第二段，作者指出对甲基苯丙胺诱发的急性精神病虽然目前没有标准的治疗方法，但常用的抗精神病药物是有效的，而在本文中，即使使用了高剂量的常用抗精神病药物，患者的症状没有缓解，直到 120 小时后随着冰毒在体内代谢完毕，患者的症状才缓解。这就是本病例的特别之处。此段我们可以看到非常经典的段落结构：第一句是引出话题，中间是举例说明，最后是总结：

Currently there are no clear guidelines for the management of acute psychosis precipitated by illicit drugs[16]. Antipsychotic medications, with or without benzodiazepines, are normally effective in standard doses and are widely used[17]. A prospective randomized study[13] administered 2 to 4 mg of lorazepam or 2.5 to 5 mg of droperidol intravenously to 166 severely agitated persons presenting to an emergency department with methamphetamine-induced acute psychosis or methamphetamine-precipitated relapse of a psychotic disorder. The patients' behavior generally settled to cooperative, somnolent, or easily roused within 30 minutes of administration of either medication. In contrast, our patient was administered standard doses of lorazepam, ziprasidone, zuclopenthixol acetate, and droperidol within the first hour, yet he remained dangerously hostile and combative (see Table 1). Other prospective randomized studies have reported that either regular olanzapine and haloperidol[18], quetiapine and haloperidol[19], or aripiprazole and risperidone[20] produce clinically significant reductions in psychotic symptomatology in cases of amphetamine-induced psychosis. Therefore, the current case is remarkable for severe psychotic agitation that was refractory to ultra-high doses of multiple antipsychotic medications and benzodiazepines（see Fig. 1 for cumulative chlorpromazine and diazepam equivalents）. The medications did not seem to alter the clinical course of his relapse. Rather, his relapse appeared to be self-limited to the clearance of the endogenous methamphetamine.

目前对于毒品诱发的急性精神病的处理尚无明确的指南[16]。抗精神病药物，无论是否含有苯二氮䓬类药物，在标准剂量下通常是有效的，并且被广泛使用[17]。一项前瞻性随机研究[13]对 166 名因甲基苯丙胺诱发的急性精神病或甲基苯丙胺诱发的精神障碍复发而到急诊科就诊的严重躁动患者静脉注射 2～4 mg 劳拉西泮或 2.5～5 mg 氟哌啶醇。患者的行为在给药 30 分钟内一般稳定，表现为合作、嗜睡或易醒。相比之下，我们的患者在第一个小时内被给予标准剂量的劳拉西泮、齐拉西酮、醋酸珠氯噻醇和氟哌啶醇，但他仍然具有危险的敌意和好斗性（见表 1）。其他前瞻性随机研究报道，无论是常规的奥氮平和氟哌啶醇[18]、喹硫平和氟哌啶醇[19]，还是阿立哌唑和利培酮[20]，在安非他明诱发的精神病病例中，都能显著减少临床精神病症状。因此，目前的病例对超高剂量的多种抗精神病药物和苯二氮䓬类药物难以治愈的严重精神病性躁动具有显著意义。这些药物似乎并没有改变他复发的临床过程。相反，复发后的好转应该是因为甲基苯丙胺代谢完了。

接下来的一段作者对治疗过程进行了回顾和分析，体现了该病例中能够得到的有用的经验（略）。作者还重点对可能的发病机制进行了探讨：

We hypothesized that our patient's poor clinical response was from a genetic polymorphism in the drug-metabolizing activity of cytochrome P450 enzymes … After he had recovered, he provided informed consent for a buccal swab of cheek cells for pharmacogenomic testing. The results of the test were two normal functioning alleles of the CYP2D6 enzyme … thus refuting our hypothesis … Benztropine has also been reported to exacerbate psychosis in persons with schizophrenia … however, this effect is controversial[25].

我们推测患者的不良临床反应来自细胞色素 P450 酶药物代谢活性的遗传多态性……康复后，他同意用口腔拭子拭取颊细胞进行药物基因组学测试。检测结果……反驳了我们的假设……据报道，苯托品也会加重精神分裂症患者的精神病……但存在争议[25]。

Degenerative changes in a patient's dopaminergic pathways may also account for a suboptimal effect of antipsychotic treatment. Chronic amphetamine abuse is known to cause enduring structural and functional changes in dopaminergic systems, which reduces the efficacy of antipsychotic medications[26] ... Of interest, our patient's father had comorbid ADHD and manic psychotic disorder, and our patient's male sibling had major depression and binge eating disorder. Taken together, this suggests a strong genetic contribution of dysfunctional dopaminergic signaling to account for our patient's psychiatric illnesses, as well as the refractory nature of his psychosis to treatment.

患者多巴胺能通路的退行性改变也可能是抗精神病药物治疗效果欠佳的原因。长期滥用安非他明会导致多巴胺能系统发生持久的结构和功能变化,从而降低抗精神病药物的疗效[26]……患者的父亲患有多动症和躁狂精神障碍,患者的兄弟患有重度抑郁症和暴食症。综上所述,这表明多巴胺能信号功能失调在很大程度上是遗传因素造成的,这可以解释此患者的精神疾病,以及他的精神疾病的难治性。

作者在"Table 1"(Medications administered to the patient in our emergency department and selected behavioral observations)和"Table 2"(Medications administered every 24 hours since presentation to our emergency department)中描述了治疗用药的时间轴。

最后作者对整个治疗过程进行了总结(采用过去时),穿插了对将来类似患者的治疗的建议(采用现在时):

Our patient experienced a particularly severe acute psychotic relapse which lasted 96 to 120 hours and was precipitated by daily cannabis and binges of crystal methamphetamine. His acute psychosis was marked by continuous severe hostility which was unusually resistant to ultra-high doses of multiple antipsychotic and benzodiazepine medications. In these treatment-refractory cases, there is a significant potential for harm to the patient, staff, and the public. Risks to the patient include self-harm, suicide, and adverse effects of medications. Although the adverse effects of psychoactive medications are difficult to monitor in uncooperative patients they can be life threatening and thus warrant special attention ...

我们的患者经历了一次特别严重的急性精神病复发,持续了 96 至 120 小时,并因每日吸食大麻和冰毒而加重。他的急性精神病以持续的严重敌意为特征,对超高剂量的多种抗精神病药物和苯二氮䓬类药物异常耐药。在这些治疗难治性病例中,对患者、工作人员和公众都有很大的潜在危害。患者面临的风险包括自残、自杀和药物副作用。虽然不合作的患者中精神活性药物的不良反应很难被监测到，但不良反应可能危及生命，因此需要特别注意……

第 2 节　回顾性研究

回顾性研究是一种回顾过去并评估已经发生的事件的研究。研究人员在项目开始时就已经知道每个受试者的结果。这些研究没有记录事件发生时的数据，而是使用参与者的回忆和与本回顾性研究无关的历史数据。因此，与必须长期跟踪受试者并在严格控制的条件下记录数据的前瞻性研究相比，回顾性研究可以更快地完成评估，而且需要的经费更少，因此非常适合年轻的临床医生，作为科学研究的起步，并锻炼自己的写作能力。回顾性研究非常适合罕见疾病，作者可以通过数据库或多中心的病例研究罕见疾病。

回顾性研究属于观察性研究。因为会引入更多的偏差和错误，回顾性不如前瞻性可靠，但在回顾性研究结果的基础上可进一步开展前瞻性研究。通过回顾性研究研究人员可以确定受试者变量（风险因素、个人特征等）与感兴趣的结果之间是否存在统计学上显著的关系。一些回顾性研究是探索性的，目的是提出令人感兴趣的假说，另一些研究则可以验证已有的假说。

回顾性研究的写作必须遵循"STROBE 声明"[5]，即"加强流行病学中观察性研究报告质量的声明"（STrengthening the Reporting of OBservational studies in Epidemiology，STROBE）。"STROBE 声明"包含了在三种主要观察性流行病学研究类型（队列研究、病例对照研究和横断面研究）中应报告的项目。我们认为，对于较多病例的案例系列报道（Case series），类似单臂的回顾性研究。2004 年 STROBE 工作组成立，同时建立了网站。

"STROBE 声明"清单由 22 个条目组成，这些条目是优质的观察性研究报告必备的重要内容（表 7.2）。18 个条目适用于所有三种研究设计，其余 4 个条目（条目 6、12、14 和 15）则根据设计类型而定。在 STROBE 网站可以获得三种设计方案相应的条目清单。

"STROBE 声明"旨在帮助作者撰写分析性观察研究报告，协助编辑和同行评审人审稿，也帮助读者严格评价已发表论文。

表 7.2　STROBE 声明:观察性研究报告中应当纳入的条目清单

	条目	建议
题目和摘要	1a	在题目或摘要中用常用术语表明研究所采用的设计
	1b	在摘要中对所做工作和获得的结果做一个简明的总结
引言		
背景/原理	2	解释研究的科学背景和原理
目的	3	阐明具体研究目的,包括任何预先设定的假设
方法		
研究设计	4	陈述研究设计的关键内容
研究设置	5	描述研究机构、研究地点及相关资料,包括招募的时间范围、暴露、随访而后数据收集等
参与者	6a	队列设计:描述纳入标准,参与者的来源和选择方法,随访方法;病例-对照设计:描述纳入标准,病例和对照的来源及确认病例和选择对照的方法,病例和对照选择的原理;横断面设计:描述纳入标准,参与者的来源和选择方法
	6b	队列设计:对于配对设计,应说明配对标准及暴露和非暴露的人数;病例-对照设计:对于配对设计,应说明配对标准和每个病例配对的对照数
变量	7	明确定义结局、暴露、预测因子、可能的混杂因素及效应因素,如果相关,给出诊断标准
数据来源/测量	8	对每个有意义的变量,给出数据来源和详细的测量方法;如果有一个以上的组,描述各组之间测量方法的可比性
偏倚	9	描述解决潜在偏倚的方法
样本大小	10	描述样本量的确定方法
定量变量	11	解释定量变量是如何分析的,如果相关,描述分组的方法和原因
统计方法	12	描述所用的所有统计方法;描述所用分析亚组和交互作用的方法;解释如何解决数据缺失;队列设计:如果相关,描述解决失访问题的方法;病例-对照设计:如果相关,描述如何对病例和对照进行配对;横断面设计:如果相关,描述抽样策略的分析方法;描述所用的灵敏度分析方法

	条目	建议
结果		
参与者	13	报告研究各阶段参与者的人数,如可能合格的人数,参与筛查的人数,证实合格的人数,纳入研究的人数,完成随访的人数及完成分析的人数; 解释在各阶段参与者退出研究的原因; 考虑使用流程图
描述性数据	14	描述参与者的特征(如人口统计学、临床和社会特征)以及暴露和潜在混杂因素的相关信息; 描述就每一个待测变量而言缺失数据的参与者人数; 队列设计:总结随访时间(如平均随访时间和全部随访时间)
结局数据	15	队列设计:报告随时间变化的事件数或综合指标 病例-对照设计:报告各种暴露类别的人数或暴露综合指标 横断面设计:报告结局事件数或综合指标
主要结果	16	报告未校正的估计值,如果相关,给出混杂因素校正后的估计值及其精确度(如 95% 可信区间);阐明按照哪些混杂因素进行了校正以及选择这些因素进行校正的原因; 如对连续变量进行分组,要报告每组观察值的范围; 对有意义的危险因素,最好把相对危险化成针对有意义的时间范围的绝对危险度
其他分析	17	如亚组分析、交互作用分析
讨论		
关键结果	18	根据研究目标概括关键结果
局限性	19	讨论研究的局限性,包括潜在偏倚或不准确的来源,讨论任何潜在偏倚的方向和大小
解释	20	结合研究目标、研究局限性、多重分析、相似研究的结果和其他相关证据,谨慎给出一个总体的结果解释
可推广性	21	讨论研究结果的普适性(外推有效性)
其他信息		
资金来源	22	提供研究资金的来源和资助机构在研究中的作用,如果相关,提供资助机构在本文基于的初始研究中的作用

从表 7.2 可以看出,回顾性研究的论文格式要求和"CONSORT 声明"大体相似。下面我们介绍一篇回顾性研究论文。论文的题目是"Outcomes of patients with limited-stage plasmablastic lymphoma：A multi-institutional retrospective study"[6]。

"INTRODUCTION"的第一段是疾病的整体介绍,包括发病率,病理特征和发病机制,相当于漏斗的最上部分。用现在时,用了 7 篇参考文献。

Plasmablastic lymphoma（PBL）is a rare subtype of non-Hodgkin Lymphoma（NHL）first recognized as a distinct clinicopathologic disease entity in 1997 by the World Health Organization classification of lymphoid neoplasms[1]. Immunohistochemistry is consistent with a plasma cell phenotype with lack of expression of typical B-cell markers, such as CD20. Both MYC translocations and EBV expression（i. e., Epstein-Barr virus encoded RNA, EBER）are commonly detected[2,3]. The clinical characteristics of patients diagnosed with PBL can be heterogenous. The diagnosis is commonly associated with immunocompromised states（e. g., human immunodeficiency virus ［HIV], solid organ transplant patients）but occurs in immunocompetent patients as well[3,4,5]. Patients infected with HIV' as well as those who are immunocompetent, commonly have extranodal involvement at presentation with the most common sites of involvement the oral cavity/jaw and GI tract[6,7].

浆母细胞淋巴瘤(PBL)是一种罕见的非霍奇金淋巴瘤(NHL)亚型,于 1997 年首次被世界卫生组织淋巴样肿瘤分类认定为一种独特的临床病理类型[1]。免疫组织化学与浆细胞表型一致,缺乏典型 B 细胞标记物(如 CD20)的表达。MYC 易位和 EBV 表达(即 Epstein-Barr 病毒编码 RNA, EBER)都是常见的检测方法[2,3]。诊断为 PBL 的患者的临床特征可能是异质性的。该诊断通常与免疫功能低下状态[例如,人类免疫缺陷病毒感染(HIV),实体器官移植患者]有关,但也发生在免疫功能正常的患者中[3,4,5]。感染 HIV 的患者,以及免疫能力强的患者,在发病时通常有结外受累,最常见的受累部位是口腔/颌和胃肠道[6,7]。

注意,"i. e."后面有逗号。此外一般中括号在小括号的里面。对于连续的参考文献的引用,通常采用连字符,如"3-5"。这个杂志的格式是例外,因此要注意。

第二段对患者的预后研究进行了介绍,相当于漏斗的中部。这里主要用一般现在时。通过采用现在完成时提示本研究将进行相关的研究。

The clinical course of PBL is characterized by an aggressive course, high relapse rates after cytotoxic chemotherapy, and poor outcomes[5,7,8,9,10,11]. Mounting data have suggested that limited-stage (LS) disease (Ann Arbor stage I - II) may have a more favorable prognosis.[7,10] However, there has yet to be a dedicated review of LS patients and treatment recommendations from prior reviews have not commonly differentiated LS from extensive-stage (ES) patients. Thus, many patients with LS disease are treated with aggressive therapy, such as auto-SCT consolidation, based on the poor outcomes of PBL patients overall[7,12,13,14]. In addition, prognostic factors (i. e., HIV status, performance status, etc.) that affect outcomes of PBL patients in certain series have never been analyzed specifically in LS patients.

PBL 的临床过程具有侵袭性,细胞毒性化疗后复发率高,预后差的特点[5,7,8,9,10,11]。越来越多的数据表明,局限期(LS)PBL(Ann Arbor I~II 期)可能有更有利的预后[7,10]。然而,目前还没有针对 LS 患者的详尽描述,并且先前综述的治疗建议并没有将 LS 患者与广泛期(ES)患者区分开来。因此,基于 PBL 患者总体预后不佳考虑,对许多 LS 患者进行了强化治疗,如自体-SCT 巩固治疗[7,12,13,14]。此外,一些病例系列报道没有对影响 LS 患者的预后因素(即 HIV、体力状态等)进行专门的分析。

最后一段描述本研究的主要内容。"We describe"是常用的开头语,采用现在时。

We describe the clinical characteristics, treatment patterns, and outcomes of LS PBL patients through a multi-center retrospective analysis to provide insights into prognosis and support clinical decision making.

我们通过多中心回顾性分析来描述 LS PBL 患者的临床特征、治疗模式和结局,以提供对预后的见解和支持临床决策。

METHODS 部分的第一段描述了时间,地点,患者诊断等数据,采用过去式。

Data on patients with LS PBL from 13 U. S. academic centers were collected. Institutional review board approval was obtained at each site and patients with a confirmed histologic diagnosis of PBL were eligible for inclusion. Determination of LS disease was determined by the Ann Arbor staging system[15]. Patients diagnosed with PBL between 1/1/1990 and 6/1/2018 were included. Baseline demographic, clinical, laboratory, pathology, and outcome data were extracted by retrospective chart review and included in a study-specific data collection spreadsheet … EBV expression of diagnostic tissue was reported as positive or negative without regard for utilization of a specific assay. Subsequently, individual centers were asked to qualify EBER expression performed on the diagnostic specimens as positive or negative if available. Responses were assessed by individual investigators utilizing institutional standard imaging modalities.

来自 13 个美国学术中心的 LS PBL 患者的数据被收集起来。每个中心都获得了机构审查委员会的批准,组织学诊断为 PBL 的患者符合入选条件。LS 疾病的判定采用 Ann Arbor 分期系统[15]。纳入 1990 年 1 月 1 日至 2018 年 6 月 1 日期间诊断为 PBL 的患者。通过回顾性图表提取基线人口统计学、临床、实验室、病理和结果数据,并将其纳入研究特定数据收集电子表格……诊断组织的 EBV 表达为阳性或阴性,任何测定方法都可。个别中心被要求对诊断标本上的 EBER 表达进行阳性或阴性鉴定。每个研究者利用本机构标准成像方式进行疗效评估。

第二段是统计学方法,这里不再赘述。如前介绍,描述具体的统计学方法用过去式,如:"Kaplan-Meier estimates were utilized for time to event analysis for overall survival (OS)"。介绍数据的描述方法用现在时,如:"The univariate and multivariate regression results are reported as hazard ratio with 95% confidence interval"。

"RESULTS" 部分的第一段用过去时介绍患者特征 (Patient characteristics),但描述表格和图的内容用现在时,如"Baseline characteristics are included in Table 1"。百分数一定要和具体病例数一起出现,如"LDH was elevated in 23.6% (17/72) of the patients"。对于超过 70% 的数据,可以用"most"来强调:

A total of 80 patients with LS PBL were identified. Baseline characteristics are included in Table 1. The median age was 58 years (range: 21~91); the male: female ratio was 4.7 : 1; and 20.5% (16/78) of the patient population were HIV positive. LDH was elevated in 23.6% (17/72) of the patients. Most patients (70.0%, or 56/80), were stage I or stage IE. Most patients, 82.5% (66/80), had extranodal involvement with the most common sites being sinus/nasopharynx 36.3% (29/80); GI tract 17.5% (14/80) including stomach, small intestine, and large intestine; along with 6.3% (5/80) occurring within the oral cavity, mandible, or tonsils (Table A1). Most patients (94.3%, or 66/70) had an ECOG PS of 0~2. Ki-67 ≥ 80% was noted in 73.1% (38/52) of patients. EBV expression was defined as positive on tumor biopsy in 72.6% (53/73) of patients. Of the 44 tumor samples that were specifically evaluated for EBER by in situ hybridization, 77.3% (34/44) were positive and 22.7% (10/44) were negative.

共有 80 例 LS PBL 患者。基线特征包含在表 1 中。中位年龄为 58 岁（范围：21~91 岁）；男女比例为 4.7∶1；20.5%（16/78）患者 HIV 阳性。23.6%（17/72）的患者 LDH 升高。大多数患者（70.0%，56/80）为 I 期或 IE 期。大多数患者[82.5%（66/80）]有结外受累，最常见的部位是鼻窦/鼻咽部[36.3%（29/80）]；胃肠道 17.5%（14/80），包括胃、小肠和大肠；6.3%（5/80）发生在口腔、下颌骨或扁桃体（表 A1）。大多数患者（94.3%，66/70）的 ECOG PS 为 0~2。73.1%（38/52）的患者 Ki-67≥80%。72.6%（53/73）的患者在肿瘤活检中 EBV 表达阳性。44 例经原位杂交特异性评价的肿瘤标本中，77.3%（34/44）阳性，22.7%（10/44）阴性。

第二段是"Patient treatment"，采用过去时。小于 10 的数字一般用单词，如"seven（8.8%）received radiation therapy"。最后一句中作者写"1（1.3%）was HIV⁺…"是不规范的。

Treatment characteristics are described in Table 2 and Figure 1. Of the 80 patients, 65 (81.3%) received frontline chemotherapy, of which 29 (36.3%) received frontline chemotherapy followed by consolidation with radiation therapy (RT), and 36 (45.0%) received frontline chemotherapy with no RT consolidation. Of the 65 patients that received frontline chemotherapy, 33 (50.8%) received EPOCH-based (…) treatment, 14 (21.5%) received a CHOP-based (…) regimen, and 11 (16.9%) received aggressive Hyper-CVAD (…) or modified Hyper-CVAD-like regimen. Of the 65 patients that received frontline chemotherapy, eight (12.3%) underwent Auto-SCT consolidation. A minority of patients, 14 (21.5%), received bortezomib and 15 (23.1%) received rituximab as part of their frontline chemotherapy regimen. Data on CD20 expression for each diagnostic sample were not available. Of the 15 patients that did not receive frontline chemotherapy, seven (8.8%) received radiation therapy (RT) alone, six (7.5%) received surgical resection alone, one (1.3%)

did not receive any therapy, and 1 (1.3%) was HIV⁺ and received anti-retroviral therapy (ART) alone.

治疗特征见表2和图1。80例患者中,65例(81.3%)患者接受一线化疗,其中29例(36.3%)患者接受一线化疗后巩固放疗(RT),36例(45.0%)患者接受一线化疗,未巩固放疗。在接受一线化疗的65名患者中,33名(50.8%)接受了EPOCH(……),14名(21.5%)接受了CHOP(……)方案,11名(16.9%)接受了积极的Hyper-CVAD(……)或改良的Hyper-CVAD样方案。在65名接受一线化疗的患者中,8名(12.3%)接受了Auto-SCT巩固治疗。少数患者中,14名(21.5%)接受硼替佐米,15名(23.1%)接受利妥昔单抗作为一线化疗方案的一部分。每个诊断样本的CD20表达数据缺乏。在未接受一线化疗的15例患者中,7例(8.8%)单独接受放射治疗(RT),6例(7.5%)单独接受手术切除,1例(1.3%)未接受任何治疗,1例(1.3%)为HIV+并只接受抗反转录病毒治疗(ART)。

第三段是治疗结局(Patient outcomes and outcomes by frontline therapy),采用过去时。先介绍基本的治疗情况:

With a median follow up of 34 months (1~196), the 3-year PFS and OS rates were 72% (95% CI 62, 83) and 79% (95% CI 70, 89), respectively (Figure 2A). Patient outcomes by frontline therapy are detailed in Table 2. The PFS and OS outcomes were investigated according to patients receiving frontline chemotherapy with consolidative RT versus frontline chemotherapy without consolidative RT (Figure 2B) as well as patients achieving a complete remission (CR) to frontline chemotherapy with consolidative RT versus patients achieving a CR who did not receive consolidative RT. Patients that received frontline chemotherapy with consolidative RT (N＝29) received a median of four cycles of chemotherapy (range 1~6), while patients who received frontline chemotherapy without RT consolidation received a median of six cycles of chemotherapy (range 1~6).

中位随访时间为34个月(1~196),3年PFS和OS率分别为72%(95% CI 62, 83)和79%(95% CI 70, 89)(图2A)。一线治疗的患者结局详见表2。对接受一线化疗合并巩固性放疗的患者与不接受巩固性放疗的一线化疗的患者(图2B)之间,以及接受巩固性放疗的一线化疗完全缓解(CR)的患者与未接受巩固性放疗的CR的患者之间的PFS和OS结果进行了比较。接受一线化疗合并巩固性放疗的患者(N＝29)接受了中位数为4个周期的化疗(范围1~6)。而接受一线化疗而未进行RT巩固的患者则接受了中位数为

6 个化疗周期(范围 1~6)。

接下去的段落是不同亚组患者的比较。这里"p-value＝0.395"的格式也是比较特殊,一般写成"$p=0.395$"。这段有个比较的句型 "… had a hazard ratio of 0.61…, relative to…"。有个比较特别的用法,即"versus"用于多个项目的比较:

The patients that received chemotherapy and consolidative RT as frontline therapy had a hazard ratio (HR) of 0.61 (95% CI, 0.19, 1.9, by univariate analysis) for PFS and 0.33 (95% CI, 0.064, 1.7) for OS, relative to patients receiving frontline chemotherapy alone. The hazard ratio reduction for progression by 39% (p-value = 0.395) and death by 67% (p-value = 0.189) were not statistically significant.

与单独接受一线化疗的患者相比,接受化疗和巩固性放疗作为一线治疗的患者,PFS 的风险比(HR)为 0.61 (95% CI 0.19,单因素分析为 1.9),OS 的风险比(HR)为 0.33 (95% CI 0.064, 1.7)。进展风险比降低 39%($p=$0.395),死亡风险比降低 67%($p=$0.189),无统计学意义。

Outcomes based on frontline therapy were analyzed according to EPOCH-based (N = 33) versus CHOP-based (N = 14) versus Hyper-CVAD based frontline therapy (N = 11) as well as patients that received Auto-SCT consolidation (N = 8) versus no Auto-SCT consolidation (N = 57) (Table 2; Figure 2C).

根据基于 EPOCH 的(N＝33)、基于 CHOP 的(N＝14)和基于 Hyper-CVAD 的一线治疗(N＝11)以及接受 Auto-SCT 巩固治疗(N＝8)和未接受 Auto-SCT 巩固治疗(N＝57)对一线治疗的结果进行分析(表 2;图 2C)。

There was a total of twenty reported patient deaths (25%). Eight deaths (10%) were attributed to PBL, three deaths (4%) attributed to toxicity (one with frontline EPOCH, one with frontline Hyper-CVAD, and one with salvage chemotherapy), and nine deaths (11%) related to other causes including sepsis not related to treatment (N = 1), secondary AML (N = 1), and not specified (N = 7).

总共报道了 20 例死亡患者(25%)。8 例死亡(10%)归因于 PBL,3 例死亡(4%)归因于药物毒性(1 例一线 EPOCH,1 例一线 Hyper-CVAD,1 例挽救性化疗),9 例死亡(11%)与其他原因相关,包括与治疗无关的败血症(N＝1)、继发性 AML (N＝1)和未记载的原因(N＝7)。

注意:"deaths"可以是复数。死亡原因可以用"attributed to"和" related

to"。

The 3-year LFS rates, excluding death by treatment related mortality (TRM) and death not attributed to PBL, for the entire cohort (N=69), for patients that received frontline chemotherapy alone (n=30), and for those receiving frontline chemo-RT (N=27) along with 3-year LFS rates (including death by TRM as an event and excluding other causes of death not attributed to PBL) for the entire cohort (N=72), for patients receiving frontline chemotherapy alone (N=33), and for patients receiving frontline chemo-RT (N=27) were analyzed (Table 2).

表 2 展现了剔除死于治疗相关死亡(TRM)和非 PBL 原因死亡的 3 年 LFS 率,包括整个队列(N=69),仅接受一线化疗治疗的病人(N=30),那些接受一线化疗-放疗(N=27)的病人。表 2 还展现了包括死于 TRM 和排除非 PBL 死亡的 3 年 LFS 率,包括整个队列(N=72),仅接受一线化疗的病人(N=33)和接受一线化疗-放疗的病人(N=27)。

Patients had PFS and OS outcomes investigated according to stage I/IE versus II/IIE (Figure 2D) and HIV⁺ status (Figure 2E). There were 13 patients that received either frontline RT alone or surgical resection alone with results reported in Table 2. One patient elected to proceed to hospice and passed away shortly after diagnosis with no therapy. One HIV positive patient with stage IE disease started on ART at diagnosis and achieved CR. This patient remained in CR at data submission, 29 months after diagnosis.

根据Ⅰ期/ⅠE vsⅡ期/ⅡE(图 2D)和 HIV+状态(图 2E)研究了病人的 PFS 和 OS 结果。13 例患者单独接受一线放疗或手术切除,结果见表 2。一名病人选择安宁疗护,但在诊断后不久便去世,没有接受任何治疗。一名 HIV 阳性的ⅠE 期患者在诊断时开始接受抗反转录病毒治疗并达到 CR。该患者在诊断后 29 个月仍处于 CR 状态。

接下来作者分析了预后因子(Prognostic factors):

Among the eight variables evaluated, frontline chemotherapy regimen (EPOCH-based vs. CHOP-based) and LDH (≥ULN vs. <ULN) were considered to include in the multivariate model for PFS based on the significance level of 0.15 for entry and for stay. Both variables were significant with a significance level of 0.05 (Figure A1). Comparing the reduced model with frontline chemotherapy and LDH versus the full model

with all eight variables, we fail to reject the reduced model（p-value = 0.717）implying that additional six predictors were not helpful to improve the fit over the reduced model. Holding LDH constant, EPOCH-based frontline chemotherapy reduced the PFS HR by a factor of 0.23 compared to CHOP（p = 0.029）, and holding frontline chemotherapy constant, LDH ⩾ ULN increased the PFS HR by a factor of 4.29（p = 0.029）.

在评估的 8 个变量中,根据 0.15 显著性水平,将一线化疗方案(基于 EPOCH vs 基于 CHOP)和 LDH(⩾ULN vs<ULN)纳入 PFS 的多变量模型中。两个变量均显著,显著性水平为 0.05(图 A1)。将一线化疗和 LDH 的简化模型与包含所有 8 个变量的完整模型进行比较,我们未能拒绝简化模型(p=0.717),这意味着额外的 6 个预测因子无助于改善简化模型的拟合。与 CHOP 相比,保持 LDH 不变,EPOCH 一线化疗使 PFS HR 降低到 0.23 倍(p=0.029),而保持一线化疗不变,LDH⩾ULN 使 PFS HR 增加了 4.29 倍(p=0.029)。

Among the eight variables, the use of EPOCH was the only variable selected by the stepwise procedure in the univariate analysis for OS. However, the p-value was 0.182, which was not statistically significant. The additional seven variables did not improve the model fit over the EPOCH-based chemotherapy only model（p-value = 0.778）.

在 8 个变量中,EPOCH 是 OS 单变量分析中采用逐步方法选出的唯一变量。然而,p 值为 0.182,无统计学意义。与仅基于 EPOCH 的化疗模型相比,新增的 7 个变量并未改善模型拟合(p=0.778)。

"DISCUSSION"的第一段对既往的治疗建议和存在的问题再次做了总结,凸显了本研究的价值。此段采用现在时,表明既往治疗建议的普适性。最后一句"To the best of our knowledge, this is the largest…"是常用句式。如果没有十分把握,或本研究的价值不是特别大,忌用"To the best of our knowledge…"。

Because of the low incidence of patients with LS PBL and corresponding lack of prospective trials, standard treatment guidelines are not clearly defined and rely on retrospective data. Due to the aggressive nature of the disease, high relapse rates, poor outcomes of PBL, and lack of reported outcomes for patients with limited stage disease, treatment recommendations generally favor aggressive regimens. Previous reviews of both LS and ES patients have shown a trend toward better outcomes with aggressive chemotherapy or consolidation with Auto-SCT[13,14] while other reviews have not shown any clear benefit with more intensive regimens[4,5,11] leaving clinicians with significant ambiguity in making treatment recommendations' especially in patients with LS disease. To the best of our knowledge, this is the largest review of LS PBL patients.

由于 LS PBL 患者的发病率较低且缺乏前瞻性试验,标准治疗指南没有明确定义,且依赖于回顾性数据。由于该疾病的侵袭性,高复发率,PBL 预后差,以及缺乏对局限期患者预后的报道,建议的治疗通常倾向于强化的方案。先前对 LS 和 ES 患者的分析显示,强化化疗或 Auto-SCT 巩固治疗有更好的结果的趋势[13,14],而其他综述没有显示更强化的方案有任何明显的益处[4,5,11],使临床医生在制定治疗建议时存在明显的模糊性,特别是对 LS 患者。据我们所知,这是对 LS PBL 患者进行的最大样本的分析。

一般来说,第一段介绍本次研究结果,但作者在第二段才对本研究进行总结:

Herein, we describe overall favorable outcomes of LS PBL with three-year PFS and OS probabilities of 72% (95% CI 62, 83) and 79% (95% CI 69, 89), respectively and a three-year LFS probability of 83% (95% CI 73, 93) when censoring for death unrelated to PBL and 86% (95% CI 78, 96) when censoring for death unrelated to PBL and for death related to TRM.

在本文中,我们描述了 LS PBL 的总体有利结果,3 年的 PFS 和 OS 率分别为 72%(95% CI,62,83)和 79%(95% CI,69,89);当删剪与 PBL 无关的死亡时,3 年的 LFS 率为 83%(95% CI,73,93),当删剪与 PBL 无关的死亡和与 TRM 相关的死亡时,LFS 概率为 86%(95% CI,78,96)。

第三段对预后因子的分析结果进行了介绍,用过去时:

In terms of clinical variables, there was no trend toward inferior PFS or OS in patients who were HIV+ at the time of diagnosis and seemed to be a trend toward improvement in PFS and OS in HIV⁺ patients in the multivariate analysis, although this was not statistically significant. Multivariate regression analysis showed a statistically significant increase in HR for PFS with elevated LDH at diagnosis when holding frontline chemotherapy constant and failed to add other clinical variables such as sex, age, stage, or EBV expression to the analysis to show any statistically significant effects on PFS or OS.

在临床变量方面,在诊断时为 HIV⁺ 的患者中,PFS 或 OS 没有较差的趋势,在多变量分析中,HIV⁺ 患者的 PFS 和 OS 似乎有改善的趋势,尽管这没有统计学意义。多因素回归分析显示,在保持一线化疗不变的情况下,诊断时 LDH 升高的 PFS 患者的 HR 有统计学意义的增加,但其他临床变量(如性别、年龄、分期或 EBV 表达)对 PFS 或 OS 没有统计学意义的影响。

第四段对本研究的不足之处进行了介绍。作者主要是做了一些理论的推测,因此用现在时。"Caution should be used (taken) when interpreting …"是常用的句式。

Caution should be used when interpreting the effect of different treatment variables on outcomes as this is a retrospective, non-randomized comparison of different subgroups of a relatively small number of patients. In addition, the rationale behind each choice of treatment (e. g., choice of frontline chemotherapy, RT consolidation, etc.) for each patient is unknown. As well, this data set does not include the number of patients with PET-CT scans and/or bone marrow biopsies at diagnosis, and it is possible some patients were more rigorously staged than others.

在解释不同治疗变量对结果的影响时应谨慎,因为这是一项对相对较少患者的不同亚组的回顾性、非随机比较。此外,每位患者选择的治疗方法(如选择一线化疗、放疗巩固等)背后的理由尚不清楚。同样,该数据集不包括诊断时进行 PET-CT 扫描和/或骨髓活检的患者数量,并且可能有些患者比其他患者分期更严格。

第五段和第六段对不同方案的疗效差异进行了分析。每次都是先用过去式描述结果,然后进行推测时用"may":

Patients that received aggressive frontline therapy, defined as Hyper-CVAD or modified Hyper-CVAD did not show improvement in PFS or OS compared to other frontline cytotoxic regimens such as CHOP- or EPOCH-based therapy. Patients that received EPOCH-based frontline therapy did show a trend towards improvement in PFS and OS compared to those that received CHOP-based frontline therapy with multivariate regression analysis showing a statistically significant improvement in PFS with EPOCH-based therapy when holding LDH constant. Any outcome improvement associated with EPOCH-versus CHOP-based frontline therapy may be related to selection bias, with fitter patients being more likely to receive EPOCH-based therapy. As well，patients treated with EPOCH-based therapy may have been more often treated in an era with improved supportive care measures as compared to CHOP-based therapy，perhaps affecting outcomes.

与其他一线细胞毒性方案(如 CHOP 或 EPOCH)相比，接受强化的一线治疗(指 Hyper-CVAD 或改良的 Hyper-CVAD)的患者在 PFS 或 OS 方面没有改善。与接受以 CHOP 为基础的一线治疗的患者相比，接受 EPOCH 为基础的一线治疗的患者确实显示出 PFS 和 OS 改善的趋势，多变量回归分析显示，在保持 LDH 不变的情况下，EPOCH 为基础的治疗的 PFS 有统计学意义的改善。EPOCH 与 CHOP 一线治疗相关的任何结果改善可能与选择偏倚有关，更健康的患者更有可能接受 EPOCH 治疗。同样，与基于 CHOP 的治疗相比，接受 EPOCH 治疗的患者可能更常在支持治疗措施改善的时代接受治疗，这可能会影响结果。

Patients that received RT consolidation after frontline therapy were associated with improvements in PFS and OS but neither was shown to be statistically significant in the multivariate regression analysis. This trend seemed to be consistent when analyzing patients that achieved a CR after receipt of frontline chemotherapy. However，data regarding disease location and disease bulk that could perhaps affect the decision for RT consolidation is not available.

一线治疗后接受放疗巩固的患者 PFS 和 OS 有改善，但在多变量回归分析中均未显示出统计学意义。在分析接受一线化疗后达到 CR 的患者时，这一趋势似乎是一致的。然而我们不知道肿瘤位置和体积是否会影响 RT 巩固治疗的采用。

最后是总结。该文的结果采用过去时，表示结果仅代表此次研究，不是一个普适的结论。"In summary, this review demonstrates …"是常用的句式，采用现在时。

In summary，this review demonstrates the favorable outcomes in PBLLS patients，especially in those able to receive definitive therapy for their disease. Aggressive frontline therapy with Hyper-CVAD based regimens or auto-SCT consolidation did not improve outcomes. Frontline therapy with EPOCH based regimens showed improved PFS outcomes versus CHOP based regimens that were statistically significant in multivariate regression analysis. Radiation consolidation after frontline chemotherapy was associated with improved outcomes over frontline chemotherapy alone，but these results did not meet statistical significance.

总之，本研究表明 PBL LS 患者预后良好，特别是那些能够接受明确治疗的患者。基于 Hyper-CVAD 方案或自体 SCT 巩固治疗的强化一线治疗并未改善预后。在多变量回归分析中，基于 EPOCH 的一线治疗方案与基于 CHOP 的方案相比，PFS 结果有所改善，具有统计学意义。一线化疗后的巩固放疗比单独一线化疗的预后更好，但结果不具有统计学意义。

"… was associated with improved outcomes over … but these results did not meet statistical significance"是常用的结果不具有统计学意义的描述。

第3节　撰写阴性结果研究论文

当研究工作产生阴性（negative）结果时，研究人员经常感到失望，这意味着要接受无效假设。研究人员通常不愿意公布阴性结果，尤其是在他们的数据不支持他们很看重的新的假设的时候。然而阴性结果对研究的进展至关重要，它告诉研究人员，他们走错了路，或者他们目前的技术无效。这是发现以前未知事物的自然而必要的一部分。

分析导致阴性结果的原因是研究人员不可或缺的一部分，同时公布正确的阴性结果有助于科学进步。很多杂志和组织也鼓励发表阴性研究结果。BioMed Central 曾经出版了《Journal of Negative Results in Biomedicine》，但很遗憾的是在 2017 年 9 月停刊了。

传统上，即使研究设计良好，结果具有足够的统计效能的阴性研究，期刊也不愿意发表。这种情况开始发生变化，尤其是在医学研究方面。不公布高质量的阴性结果研究对科学界和支持它的人（包括纳税人）来说是一种伤害，因为其他科学家可能会重复这项工作。对于医学研究，如果不发表和目前观点相矛盾的研究会导致目前治疗方法（可能无效）的继续使用，对病人和社会不利。

产生阴性结果的主要原因有三个：

* 最初的假设是错误的；

* 参照的研究无法复制；

* 方法问题。

临床研究试验失败的其他原因包括研究的统计效能（样本量太小）不足[7]，研究药物处置不当（如没有严格低温运输和保存）和患者脱落太多等。

大多数研究人员倾向于解决技术问题之前不展示阴性研究。在专业大会上介绍他们的工作有助于解决一些问题。在会议上发言时应该清楚地描述你的总体研究目标以及为什么它很重要，初步的结果，直截了当地说出你的困难和当前的问题。利用参会专家的集体专业知识增加帮助你找到解决方案的机会。在查阅相关文献时尽可能彻底，以找到最有前途的技术问题解决方案。在投稿时表明你仔细考虑了各种可能性，并制定了一个更好的计划。这将有助于审稿人对你的努力给予好评，甚至帮助你。

明显的技术问题的研究不适合发表论文。对于有疗效趋势，但因为样本量太小的阴性结果研究，可以尝试投稿。论文中可以这样写：

➢ To resolve this problem, it would be advisable to increase the sample size, and then…

➢ To resolve this problem, we are currently enrolling more patients to determine…

对于和最初的假设不吻合的阴性结果的研究，研究人员应该坦然对待。毕竟如果我们已经知道每个可能问题的答案，研究就没有必要了。应该重新考虑现有数据、阅读相关文献并与同事协商后提出新的假设。当然，有些研究是不可能重复，如某个正在或已经消失的流行病的相关研究。

事实上，为了鼓励发表，有学者建议不要用"negative"来描述预期结果不一致的研究，而应该采用"unsuccessful""underpowered"或"inconclusive"。毕竟"negative"在描写研究结果时属于英文中是贬义词（pejorative）[8]。

对于统计学上的阴性结果，有一种方法是用"trend"（差异大小和 95% 置信区间）代替阴性结果，弱化 p 值[9]。但这种做法没有得到学术界的普遍认可。

撰写阴性结果的临床研究论文的时候，引言、材料和方法、结果部分和阳性结果的论文没有差异，但讨论部分差异比较大。在引言中也可以让读者为阴性结果做好准备，如指出和过去的研究或假设不一致。

这里我们以《JAMA》杂志上发表的一篇论文为例看看阴性结果的研究如何撰写前言和讨论。论文的题目是"Ziritaxestat, a Novel Autotaxin Inhibitor, and Lung Function in Idiopathic Pulmonary Fibrosis: The ISABELA 1 and 2 Randomized Clinical Trials"[10]。

前言的第一段是漏斗的上部，最宽泛，介绍了特发性肺纤维化的特点、治疗方法的局限性。最后一句"here remains a major unmet need for more effective, better tolerated IPF treatments"是一个转折句，有承上启下的作用。这段用现在时，因为这些内容是公认的知识。

Idiopathic pulmonary fibrosis (IPF) is a chronic lung disease associated with progressive and irreversible fibrosis, dyspnea, lung function decline, and loss of quality of life. The median survival without treatment is approximately 3 years, with respiratory failure being the most frequent cause of death. Even though treatment with pirfenidone or nintedanib slows disease progression, patients continue to experience a loss of lung function and premature death. Furthermore, pirfenidone and nintedanib are associated with adverse effects in a substantial proportion of patients, which may lead to treatment discontinuation. Thus, there remains a major unmet need for more effective, better tolerated IPF treatments.

特发性肺纤维化(IPF)是一种与进行性和不可逆性纤维化、呼吸困难、肺功能下降和生活质量丧失有关的慢性肺病。未经治疗的中位生存期约为 3 年,其中呼吸衰竭是最常见的死亡原因。尽管吡非尼酮或宁替达尼治疗可以减缓疾病进展,但患者仍会经历肺功能丧失和过早死亡。此外,吡非尼酮和宁替达尼在很大一部分患者中与不良反应有关,这可能导致治疗中断。因此,对更有效、耐受性更好的 IPF 治疗的需求仍未得到满足。

第二段引出了溶血磷脂酸和 Autotaxin 蛋白,这是一个具体的研究领域,属于漏斗的中部。这段用的也是现在时,介绍公认的发病机制。

Pulmonary fibrosis in patients with IPF is believed to develop when aberrant responses to lung injury, including epithelial apoptosis and fibroblast recruitment, occur. Lysophosphatidic acid is thought to be at least partially responsible for mediating such responses. Autotaxin, an enzyme involved in the production of lysophosphatidic acid, is upregulated in patients with IPF and is therefore a potential target for novel IPF therapies.

IPF 患者的肺纤维化被认为是在对肺损伤的异常反应发生时发生的,包括上皮细胞凋亡和成纤维细胞募集。溶血磷脂酸至少部分负责介导这种反应。Autotaxin 蛋白是一种参与溶血磷脂酸产生的酶,在 IPF 患者中上调,因此是 IPF 新型治疗药物的潜在靶点。

第三段具体介绍了针对以上机制的一个具体药物 Ziritaxestat,因此处于漏斗的下部。这段介绍了有关 Ziritaxestat 的多个研究结果,用了过去式。

Ziritaxestat is a small-molecule, selective autotaxin inhibitor that showed promising results in a phase 2a study including 23 patients with

IPF. Ziritaxestat was well tolerated and those treated with ziritaxestat demonstrated a smaller mean change from baseline in forced vital capacity (FVC) at week 12 vs placebo. Furthermore, ziritaxestat reduced the concentration of plasma lysophosphatidic acid, with a maximum reduction from baseline of approximately 90％, confirming target engagement.

Ziritaxestat 是一种小分子选择性 autotaxin 抑制剂,在包括 23 名 IPF 患者的 2a 期研究中显示出有希望的结果。Ziritaxestat 耐受性良好,与安慰剂相比,接受 Ziritaxestat 治疗的患者在第 12 周的强迫肺活量(FVC)与基线相比平均变化较小。此外 Ziritaxestat 降低了血浆溶血磷脂酸的浓度,与基线相比最大降低了约 90％,证实针对了靶点。

在第三段的基础上很自然地引出了本研究的目的,即大样本的 3 期临床研究。按照美国 FDA 的法规,新药研究必须开展 2 个关键性的 3 期临床研究,证明结果的可重复性,因此这篇文章同时介绍了 2 个 3 期临床研究的结果。

To further evaluate the efficacy and safety of ziritaxestat for the treatment of IPF, 2 identically designed, phase 3, randomized clinical trials, ISABELA 1 and ISABELA 2, were conducted.

为了进一步评估 ziritaxestat 治疗 IPF 的疗效和安全性,进行了 2 项设计相同的 3 期随机临床试验,即 ISABELA 1 和 ISABELA 2。

讨论的第一段是研究的总结。这里用的是过去式。注意,总结一般不要用具体的数字。

In the ISABELA 1 and ISABELA 2 trials, ziritaxestat did not lead to a reduction in the annual rate of decline for FVC vs placebo; thus, the primary outcome was not met. Ziritaxestat also failed to show benefit in any of the secondary efficacy outcomes (time to first respiratory-related hospitalization, time to first respiratory-related mortality, time to first all-cause mortality or respiratory-related hospitalization, time to first acute IPF exacerbation, SGRQ total score, or distance on 6-minute walk test). All-cause mortality data showed a higher proportion of deaths with those taking 600 mg of ziritaxestat than with placebo in ISABELA 1, and a higher proportion of deaths with each ziritaxestat dose than with placebo in ISABELA 2.

在 ISABELA 1 和 ISABELA 2 试验中,与安慰剂相比,ziritaxestat 并未导致 FVC 的年下降率降低;因此,没有达到最初的结果。Ziritaxestat 在任何次要疗效结果(首次呼吸相关住院时间、首次呼吸相关死亡率、首次全因死亡率或呼吸相关住院治疗时间、首次急性 IPF 恶化时间、SGRQ 总分或 6 分钟步行距离测试)中也未显示出益处。全因死亡率数据显示,在 ISABELA 1 中,服用 600 mg Ziritaxestat 的患者的死亡比例高于安慰剂组,在 ISABALA 2 中,服用每种剂量的 Ziritaxestat 的死亡比例均高于安慰剂组。

第二段开始对结果进行解析。第二段主要是排查可能的影响因素。

Ziritaxestat did not reduce FVC decline compared with placebo, unlike in the prior phase 2a study, although the latter included a limited number of patients. As in the phase 2a study, decreases in lysophosphatidic acid were observed after ziritaxestat dosing; therefore, lack of target engagement is not considered the reason for the absence of effect on the clinical outcomes. It is unknown why the positive results of the prior phase 2a study were not replicated in the ISBAELA trials, but the limitations associated with early phase trials such as small sample sizes, short duration, and limited use of standard of care therapies may be contributing factors.

与安慰剂相比,Ziritaxestat 并没有减少 FVC 的下降,这与之前的 2a 期研究不同,尽管后者包括的患者数量有限。与 2a 期研究一样,给药后观察到溶血磷脂酸减少;因此,对临床结果没有影响的原因不是因为脱靶。目前尚不清楚为什么之前 2a 期研究的阳性结果没有在 ISBAELA 试验中复制,但与早期试验相关的局限性有关,包括样本量小、持续时间短和患者没有完全接受标准治疗。

注意这段的时态。在第二句和第三句,同一句中描述事件的动词用过去式,描述推论的动词用现在时。

第三段继续排除阴性结果的原因:

Lung function in patients receiving standard of care therapies was expected to decline at a slower rate than in untreated patients; however, this was not the case in the 2 ISABELA trials. The extent of FVC decline in the ISABELA trials differed between type of standrd of care therapy and was greatest in patients taking pirfenidone. Even though suboptimal pirfenidone dosing was observed in some patients, it was not overly frequent, and is not thought to explain the apparent worsening of lung function. In addition, phase 1 data show ziritaxestat does not affect pirfenidone concentration. Therefore, the reason for this finding remains unclear.

接受标准治疗的患者的肺功能下降速度预计低于未经治疗的患者；然而，ISABELA 的两次审判并非如此。ISABELA 试验中 FVC 下降的程度因不同类型的标准护理治疗而异，在服用吡非尼酮的患者中下降幅度最大。尽管在一些患者中吡非尼酮给药次数没有达到要求，但只是偏少，不可能是肺功能明显恶化的原因。此外，1 期数据显示齐利他司他不会影响吡非尼酮的浓度。因此，这一发现的原因尚不清楚。

类似第二段，第三段同一句中描述事件的动词用过去式，描述推论和结论的动词用现在时。

第四段继续排除影响因素：

Unlike for pirfenidone, phase 1 studies show ziritaxestat increases plasma levels of nintedanib. An increase in nintedanib levels could have led to the higher proportion of dose reductions, dose interruptions, and nondiarrheal TEAEs observed with nintedanib vs pirfenidone in the 600 mg of ziritaxestat group in the ISABELA trials. However, the dose of nintedanib administered has been shown to predict risk of diarrhea (this was the most frequent TEAE in the 600 mg of ziritaxestat group) better than plasma exposure. In the prior phase 2a study, ziritaxestat was administered as monotherapy and treatment with nintedanib was prohibited, reducing the probability of dose reductions or treatment interruptions due to interactions between drugs.

与吡非尼酮不同的是，1 期研究显示 Ziritaxestat 可提高血浆中宁替达尼的水平。在 ISABELA 试验中，600 mg Ziritaxestat 齐利他司他组中，与吡非尼酮相比，尼替达尼水平的增加可能导致剂量减少、剂量中断和非腹泻性 TEAE 的比例更高。然而，与血浆暴露相比，服用尼替达尼的剂量可以更好地预测腹泻风险（这是 600 mg Ziritaxestat 组中最常见的 TEAE）。在之前的 2a 期研究中，Ziritaxestat 作为单一疗法服用，禁止同时使用尼替达尼布治疗，降低了由于药物之间的相互作用而导致的剂量减少或治疗中断的概率。

第五段介绍了入组患者的情况，并继续解析阴性结果，即是否和种族有关：

As stated, the independent data and safety monitoring committee's recommendation to terminate the ISABELA trials was based on both a lack of efficacy and a perceived increased mortality risk. Pooled data from both ISABELA trials showed an all-cause mortality rate of 8.9% with 600 mg of ziritaxestat, 7.0% with 200 mg of ziritaxestat, and 5.5% with *placebo over a study duration of longer than 100 weeks. A greater proportion of patient deaths occurred with 600 mg of ziritaxestat than with placebo in ISABELA 1, and there was a greater proportion of patient deaths with both ziritaxestat doses vs placebo in ISABELA 2. At the time of trial termination, the number of patients enrolled and the number of patient-years of study drug exposure were greater in ISABELA 2 than in ISABELA 1. Compared with ISABELA 1, there was a greater proportion of Asian patients in ISABELA 2. Whether this <u>contributed</u> to the greater proportion of deaths (including COVID-19-related deaths) in ISABELA 2 <u>requires</u> greater understanding of regional and racial differences in patients with IPF.*

如前所述,独立数据和安全监测委员会终止 ISABELA 试验的建议是基于缺乏疗效和死亡风险增加。ISABELA 两项试验的汇总数据显示,在超过 100 周的研究时间内,600 mg Ziritaxestat 组的全因死亡率为 8.9%,200 mg 组为 7.0%,安慰剂组为 5.5%。在 ISABELA 1 中,600 mg Ziritaxestat 与安慰剂相比,患者死亡的比例更高,在 ISABELA 2 中,两种剂量的 Ziritaxestat 与安慰剂的患者死亡比例更高。在试验终止时,ISABELA 2 的入选患者数量和研究药物暴露的患者年数大于 ISABELA 1。与 ISABELA 1 相比,ISABELA 2 的亚裔患者比例更高。这是否导致 ISABELA 2 中死亡(包括新冠感染相关死亡)的比例增加,需要对 IPF 患者的地区和种族差异有更深入的了解。

最后一句对未来的建议(Require)用了现在时。

第六段对新冠流行导致的数据缺失进行了解析。这段采用过去式,但 "which <u>mitigates</u> the effect of some missing data" 是统计学知识,采用现在时。

The COVID-19 pandemic, which arose after the trials were initiated, had some effect on study conduct and resulted in many clinic-based visits being missed by patients. Study safety was ensured by permitting telephone visits in place of scheduled clinic visits and performance of blood safety assessments in local laboratories. The proportion of COVID-19-related deaths was low. When these COVID-19-related deaths occurred, they disproportionally affected patients in the ziritaxestat treatment groups. A limited proportion of patients had missing spirometry data (1% had no FVC data after the baseline assessment), which arguably did not affect the *analyses, and in addition, a mixed model for repeated measures was used, which <u>mitigates</u> the effect of some missing data.*

试验开始后出现的新冠感染大流行对研究行为产生了一些影响,导致许多患者错过了临床就诊。经过批准采用电话随访代替预定的诊所随访和在当地实验室进行血液安全评估确保了研究安全。新冠肺炎相关死亡的比例很低。当这些与新冠感染相关的死亡发生时,它们对 Ziritaxestat 治疗组的患者产生了不成比例的影响。少量患者缺乏肺活量测定数据(1%的患者在基线评估后没有 FVC 数据),这不会影响分析,此外,使用了重复测量的混合模型,这减轻了一些缺失数据的影响。

第七段从基础用药对研究的可能影响的角度解析阴性结果。这段大部分是推测,因此用现在时。

Despite the regulatory requirement, testing new IPF medications when the patient is taking a standard of care therapy is challenging because lung function is likely to decline at a slower rate than in untreated patients; however, as noted, this was not the case in the ISABELA trials. Furthermore, variability among individual patients may be amplified when testing a new therapy if the patient is taking a standard of care therapy, which can make data interpretation challenging.

尽管有监管要求,但当患者接受标准治疗时,评价新的 IPF 药物是具有挑战性的,因为肺功能的下降速度可能比未经治疗的患者慢;然而,如前所述,ISABELA 试验的情况并非如此。此外,如果患者正在接受标准治疗,那么在评价新疗法时个体患者之间的变异性可能会被放大,这可能会使数据解释变得具有挑战性。

第八段对未来的研究提出一些建议,用现在时:

Although the design of the ISABELA trials is not considered to have contributed to the negative findings, possible considerations for future IPF studies (which may increase the likelihood of identifying treatment effects) include using adaptive designs with a bayesian approach and using biomarker-based enrichment strategies with prognostic biomarkers of early or more rapid disease progression. Knowledge of patients' prior change in lung function would also allow better understanding of the rate of decline after the introduction of therapy. Even though the ISABELA trials failed, they demonstrate the potential value of observing data for 52 weeks or longer and provide information regarding the utility of different clinical outcomes. In addition, information collected during the trials, such as the faster than anticipated rate of decline for FVC in the patients taking standard of care therapy, adverse events associated with standard of care, and treatment patterns (eg, the proportion of patients switching or initiating standard of care therapy during the trials), may help inform the design of future IPF studies.

尽管 ISABELA 试验的设计没有被认为是导致负面结果的原因,但未来 IPF 研究的可能考虑因素(这可能会增加识别治疗效果的可能性)包括使用贝叶斯方法的自适应设计,以及使用基于生物标志物的富集策略和早期或更快疾病进展的预后生物标志物。了解患者先前的肺功能变化也可以更好地了解引入治疗后的下降率。尽管 ISABELA 试验失败了,但它们证明了 52 周或更长时间观察数据的潜在价值,并提供了有关不同临床结果效用的信息。此外,试验期间收集的信息,如接受标准治疗的患者的 FVC 下降速度快于预期,与标准治疗相关的不良事件,以及治疗模式(例如,试验期间转换或启动标准疗法的患者比例),可能有助于为未来 IPF 研究的设计提供信息。

第九段建议通过对类似的研究进行了分析寻找寻找本研究失败的原因。

Further investigation is needed to determine why the ISABELA trials failed. This may be determined by ongoing studies of other autotaxin inhibitors with different pharmacological characteristics to those of ziritaxestat (such as BBT-87723) or lysophosphatidic acid receptor antagonists (such as BMS-98627824). Of note, the lysophosphatidic acid receptor antagonist BMS-986020 was discontinued due to hepatobiliary toxicity; however, this was found to be unrelated to lysophosphatidic acid antagonism and, indeed, no such safety issues were identified in the ISABELA trials.

需要进一步研究以确定 ISABELA 试验失败的原因。这可以通过正在进行的对其他具有与 Ziritaxestat(如 BBT－87723)或溶血磷脂酸受体拮抗剂(如 BMS－98627824)不同药理学特征的 autotaxin 抑制剂的研究来确定。值得注意的是,溶血磷脂酸受体拮抗剂 BMS－986020 因肝胆毒性而停用;然而这与溶血磷脂酸拮抗作用无关,事实上,ISABELA 试验中没有发现此类安全性问题。

第十段是研究的局限性。注意,推测性的句子用现在时。描述发生了的事件的动作用过去式。

Limitations

There are several limitations to the 2 trials. First, the early termination of the trials is considered a possible limitation because it may have reduced the ability to adequately interpret the effect of treatment on the primary outcome. Second, enrollment in the ISABELA 1 trial was not complete so fewer patients entered the trial than planned and the outcomes beyond week 52 were not captured for all patients. Third, there were missing data or unattended study visits due to the COVID - 19 pandemic. Fourth, the COVID - 19 pandemic also may have influenced trial participation, and therefore the patient population may not reflect those participating in prior IPF trials. Fifth, the ISABELA trials were not powered to assess true differences among standard of care treatments (nintedanib vs pirfenidone vs no standard of care treatment).

局限性

这两项试验有几个局限性。第一，提前终止试验被认为是一个可能的限制，因为这可能降低了充分解释治疗对主要结果影响的能力。第二，ISABELA 1 试验的入组尚未完成，因此参加试验的患者比计划的要少，并且没有记录到所有患者在第 52 周之后的结果。第三，由于新冠感染大流行，有数据丢失和随访缺失。第四，新冠感染大流行也可能影响试验参与，因此患者人数可能和先前参与 IPF 试验的人有差异。第五，ISABELA 试验无法评估标准治疗之间的真实差异（宁替达尼、吡非尼酮与无标准治疗）。

最后是结论。对于阴性结果，结论趋向于体现此次研究，因此用过去式。

Conclusions

Ziritaxestat did not improve clinical outcomes compared with placebo in patients with IPF receiving standard of care treatment with pirfenidone or nintedanib or in those not receiving standard of care treatment.

结论

与安慰剂相比，在接受吡非尼酮或宁替达尼标准治疗的 IPF 患者或未接受标准治疗患者中，Ziritaxestat 没有改善临床结果。

总之，对于假设合理、设计完善的临床研究，即使出现阴性研究结果，不应该也要放弃发表论文的机会。

参考文献

[1] Gottlieb G J, Ragaz A, Vogel J V, et al. A preliminary communication on extensively disseminated Kaposi's sarcoma in young homosexual men[J]. The American Journal of Dermatopathology, 1981, 3(2): 111-114.

[2] Case Report Guidelines[EB/OL]. https://www.care-statement.org.

[3] Dwyer L J, Singhal N, Yu B, et al. Successful osimertinib rechallenge after relapse following adjuvant osimertinib: A case report[J]. Journal of Thoracic Oncology: Official Publication of the International Association for the Study of Lung Cancer, 2024, 19(4): 650-652.

[4] Tucker M G, Kekulawala S, Kent M, et al. Polysubstance-induced relapse of schizoaffective disorder refractory to high-dose antipsychotic medications: A case report[J]. Journal of Medical Case Reports, 2016, 10(1): 242.

[5] Strengthening the reporting of observational studies in epidemiology [EB/OL]. https://www.strobe-statement.org.

[6] Hess B T, Giri A, Park Y, et al. Outcomes of patients with limited-stage plasmablastic lymphoma: A multi-institutional retrospective study [J]. American Journal of Hematology, 2023, 98(2): 300-308.

[7] Lynch M, Moulin D, Perez J. Methadone vs. morphine SR for treatment of neuropathic pain: A randomized controlled trial and the challenges in recruitment [J]. Canadian Journal of Pain = Revue Canadienne De La Douleur, 2019, 3(1): 180-189.

[8] http://www.forbes.com/sites/henrymiller/2013/04/03/what-we-learn-can-learn-from-negative-clinical-trials/.

[9] Nead K T, Wehner M R, Mitra N. The use of "trend" statements to describe statistically nonsignificant results in the oncology literature[J]. JAMA Oncology, 2018, 4(12): 1778-1779.

[10] Maher T M, Ford P, Brown K K, et al. Ziritaxestat, a Novel Autotaxin Inhibitor, and Lung Function in Idiopathic Pulmonary Fibrosis: The ISABELA 1 and 2 Randomized Clinical Trials [J]. JAMA, 2023, 329(18): 1567-1578.

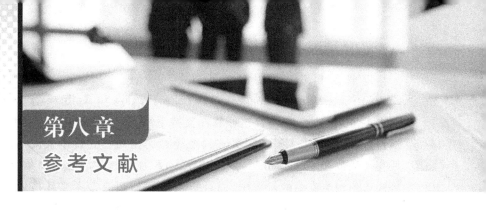

科学是在其他人的工作的基础上向前发展的，因此引用（Cite,Citation）以前的工作来表明你熟悉相关领域、说明你的思路来源、支持你的假设、肯定他人的工作以及避免剽窃误会是很重要的。参考文献可以引导读者找到和本论文相同或分歧的结果或观点，指出本论文相关数据的来源，在认可他人的工作的同时，事实上也支持了自己的研究的新颖性和价值。

第1节　参考文献的组织

一般来说，诸如"the literature suggest that …"或"there is general agreement that…"之类的陈述应有 1～2 个参考文献支持，一般不要超过 3 个。相反，一个领域的共同知识（例如人体有多少块骨骼）通常无需提供参考。文章不同部分的参考文献数量建议见表 8.1。

表 8.1　不同部分的引文的功能和的适当参考文献数量

文章部分	引文的功能	建议篇数
前言	• 介绍与研究问题相关的当前知识 • 显示以前是如何研究该问题的 • 介绍与研究问题相关的概念和变量	15～20
材料和方法	• 介绍已发布的方法、方案或标准 • 研究中使用的诊断标准的来源 • 描述复杂或鲜为人知的统计分析方法 • 样本量计算的依据 • 支持选用的研究设计或方法的合理性	5～10
结果	一般不用	0
讨论	• 支持对结果和结论的解释 • 将研究结果与其他研究结果进行比较 • 反映当前对疑问/问题的看法（争议、冲突或共识） • 支持为什么研究结果有重大意义 • 支持研究的亮点	15～20

以前参考文献的组织是耗时的。目前采用参考文献管理软件,如EndNote、Reference Manager、RefWorks、ProCite 和 Refbase 等,大大减轻了组织参考文献的工作量。这些软件支持下载、存储和组织任何类型的参考文献,包括科学论文、书籍、网页和其他类型的出版物。具体来说,这些管理软件支持从数据库(如 PubMed)自动导入,添加到软件的参考文献可以很容易地插入到论文需要的位置中,而且提供各种期刊的参考文献格式,自动格式化文内参考文献标注格式和参考文献列表。在修改论文的时候,当参考文献的内容被移动或删除的时候,管理软件将重新排列参考。引用已被接受但尚未发表的论文时会被标记为"in press"(出版中)。

自 2000 年以来,CrossRef 为各种出版物分配了数字对象标识符(Digital object identifier,DOI)。DOI 得到了出版商的一致认可。任何文献的 DOI 是永久的,而不管其在网络上的位置或 URL 是否有更改。可通过 www.crossref. org 搜索 DOI。

第 2 节　如何引用参考文献

文献引用虽然很重要,却往往是论文稿中最不受注意的方面。引文错误,包括误用和参考文献的文字(Bibliography)错误,是医学论文中常见的错误。不准确的引文会影响审稿人,误导读者,甚至传播错误知识。参考文献的文字错误还会导致影响因子的计算不精确。

引文一般可以通过直接引用(Direct quoting)、释义(Paraphrasing)或提供摘要的方法进行引用。直接引用一般是指抄录原文中超过六个以上连续的单词。直接引用可以采用引号或斜体的方法注明;每个单词和标点符号都应与原文完全相同。

直接引用一般较少,主要用于以下情况:

• 原文的表达方法非常独特。

• 原文非常简洁。

• 原文是广为人知的结论性陈述,体现特定的历史背景。

引用的时候要注意:

• 英式英语采用单引号,即:' ',美式英语采用双引号,即:" "。

• 巢式引用(nested quotes),英式英语单引号在外,即:'…"…"…';美式英语采用双引号在外,即:"… '…'…"。

- 中间有省略的时候,用三点标识即:…,ellipsis。

- 中间如果有插入作者本人的注解,用[]表示。

- 中间有用斜体来作为强调的时候,要用'my italics'注明是作者改的。

- 超过 25 个单词的引用一般单独一段,不用引号。

释义是最常用的引用方式。在释义过程中,作者用自己的语言表达他人的描述,然后注明参考文献。在解释他人的研究结果或想法的时候,作者应确认其陈述是否准确、公正。使用同义词(Synonym)和重新措辞(Rephrasing)是改变原始陈述的典型方式。释义如果包含多个句子,只在第一句标注参考文献。但如果是多个段落,则每段都要引用。如果同一个释义的不同句子出现在不同的段落中,则每个句子都要标注参考文献。

释义在措辞、语法和结构上不能与原文过于接近,否则视为"patchwriting",即"对复制的原材料进行微小更改和替换的行为('Patchwriting' refers to the act of making small changes and substitutions to copied source material—Merriam-Webster Dictionary)"。

"Patchwriting"这个词是写作教授丽贝卡·摩尔·霍华德(Rebecca Moore Howard)创造的。在 1993 年的一篇文章中她提出了以下定义:

Copying from a source text and then deleting some words, altering grammatical structures, or plugging in one-for-one synonym-substitutes.

从源文本中复制,然后删除一些单词,改变语法结构,或者插入一对一的同义词替代词。

在介绍他人研究的概要时,可以使用中性、拉近或疏远的态度对论文、书籍或章节的观点进行陈述;在拉近或疏远的方法中,不仅总结了现有的知识,而且作者也提出了自己的立场/观点。作者需要使用适当的动词准确、有说服力地表达他们的方法。对于中性总结,建议使用"comment","explain","indicate","note","describe","observe","remark","state"和"find"。一般使用现在时态表示来源是最近的并且仍然是对的结论,过去时态表示来源较旧并且可能已经过时的研究。

第 3 节　参考文献格式

每个正文中引用的文献都应在参考文献列表中,除非是"个人通信"和"未发布数据",这些数据在正文中引用,但不出现在列表中。反过来,所有的参考文献一定要在正文中有被引用。

参考文献列表中提供的信息应准确完整，以确保读者能够找到相应的文献。参考文献列表的准确性体现了作者和研究本身的可信度。为了提高准确性，ICMJE 建议"参考文献应使用电子数据库（如 PubMed）或原始文献进行验证"。参考文献的错误通常是由于抄袭了他人论文中的错误的参考文献而引起的。因此作者不应该从他人论文的参考文献列表中直接复制，必须在期刊网站或数据库上对原始论文进行确认。

大体上，杂志采用了三种参考文献格式：① 连续编号系统（Consecutive-numbering system），即众所周知的温哥华格式（Vancouver）；② 作者姓名出版年份系统（哈佛格式）；③ 脚注/尾注系统（页面底部或论文末尾，其中上标中的文献标识数字在整个论文中连续）。前两种通常用于医学，而第三种最常用于人文学科。其他不太常见的参考文献格式包括现代语言协会（MLA）、美国心理协会（APA）、芝加哥格式手册（CMS）和美国医学协会（AMA）系统。

1979 年，温哥华小组和美国国家医学图书馆（NLM）正式采用了医学文献参考的第一种格式。温哥华小组是 1978 年在不列颠哥伦比亚省温哥华举行非正式会议的医学期刊编辑小组，目的是制定期刊稿件格式指南；该小组最后发展为 ICMJE，并制定了生物医学期刊稿件要求（见 http://www.icmje.org）。这就是温哥华格式的来源。根据温哥华格式，参考文献按正文中首次提及的顺序连续编号；正文、表格和图例中的参考文献使用括号中的阿拉伯数字标识。PubMed 和 MEDLINE 采用温哥华格式。

尽管大多数生物医学期刊都采用了温哥华格式，但仍有一些更喜欢哈佛格式，因为他们倾向在阅读文章的时候同时了解文章引用了哪些作者。哈佛格式的弊端是读者如果需要在正文中查找某个参考文献被引用的位置时比较费时间，除非使用软件的查找功能。此外，当正文某个段落需要引用比较多的参考文献时，会不时中断正文。

虽然有些医学期刊采用了温哥华或哈佛格式，但可能会做一些小修改，创建了独特的引用样式。因此写作者应仔细查阅并遵循目标期刊的参考文献格式。

第 4 节　参考文献的正确使用

参考文献的引用过程要注意两个问题：一是选择合适的文献；二是以准确、合乎道德的方法引用文献。恰当的引用还会提高论文的科学档次和可读性。总体来说，在备选的文献中，应选择最相关和最新的文献，以及对本研究领域有重大贡献的文献。

最好的参考文献是同行评议的期刊发表的原始研究论文,文献综述则不能体现对完成原始研究的作者的尊重。为了更有效地总结先前的研究问题可以引用综述,并明确参考文献是综述,以避免对研究结论原创性的误导。

尽量不用或少用学生的毕业论文、会议论文、未发表的数据、摘要和个人通信,除非它们包含其他来源无法获得的重要信息。引用已被接受但尚未发表的文章时,应注明"正在印刷(in press)"或"即将出版(forthcoming)"。如果引用了"未公开资料",包括已投稿但尚未被录用的稿件中的信息时,应在文中注明"unpublished observations"或"personal communication",并注明已获得信息提供者的书面同意。除了描述理论或方法原理外,一般不引用教科书的内容。

有些文章发表后由于某些原因被撤回了,因此作者要负责检查引用的参考文献是否被撤回。为此,必须通过数据库或原始论文的杂志官网确认每篇论文的准确性,否则可能带来不好的影响。

第5节　引文的准确性与伦理

准确的文献引用使读者能够更好地了解作者的观点,并确保所传播科学的完整性,因此作者应该检查原文以核实事实。在解释或总结参考文献时应认真阅读原文,确保原作者的意图或含义没有被改变和被误解。

引用要客观,不能过度自引。自引,即论文中引用自己已经发表的论文,是一种常见做法,代表了研究过程的连续性和累积性。然而不相关的自引或过度自引是不道德的做法,而且影响论文的准确性。

避免虚假引用(Spurious citation),即引用无关的参考文献或多余的引用(如一篇参考文献即可的情况下增加不必要的参考文献)。

引用不能有偏向。偏向性引用指过多引用偏好的作者的论文和特意引用可能的审稿人的论文,而对竞争对手或不友好的作者应该被引用的论文视而不见,以及不引用对自己的研究结论不利的论文。

下面是一些常见的文献引用错误:

• 正文显示有参考文献,但文献列表中没有。

• 期刊文章作者、标题、期刊名称的拼写错误,作者姓氏和名字的颠倒,重复参考文献,缺少页码,多种参考文献格式并存,参考文献格式不符合杂志要求。

• 引用掠夺性杂志(Predatory journal)的论文。

• 书籍没有注明编辑、没有注明版本、缺少页码或章节作者（引用书籍章节时）、缺少书籍的子标题、出版商和印刷商之间的混淆、出版地点的混淆。

引文不仅是一种技术实践，也是一种修辞实践，作者通过采用不同的词汇，可以表达自己不同的态度和观点，因此必须对某一领域的文献有深入的了解。

虽然通常认为文献综述应该是"客观的"，不要采取任何立场，但也不完全如此，原因有二。其一，有时候我们需要批判性总结（Critical summary）。好的文献综述通常包含了作者对过去的知识的质量和可靠性的观点和过去的知识的立场。其二，即使我们的目标是简单的总结，也很难实现完全中立的表达，个人的感情色彩总是有的。这些色彩作者自己都有可能几乎没有注意到。如：

> **Mike describes** how hypertension impairs kidney function.
> **Mike discovered** that hypertension impairs kidney function.
> **Mike claims** hypertension impairs kidney function.

第一个动词"describes'"是中性的：看不出作者对"Mike"对该领域贡献的知识的立场。第二个动词"discovered"表示作者同意"Mike"的立场，而第三个动词"claims"则表示作者与"Mike"的观点有距离。当然同一个词的意义和上下文有关，如"suggest"可以用来表示中立或疏远。

第 6 节　原始文献和间接文献

引用原始文献，不用间接文献。原始文献（Primary source）指原创研究首次报道的文献，间接文献（或称二手文献，Secondary source）是指引用了原始文献的文献。当我们在一篇文章中（包括综述）中读到的信息来自原始文献的时候，如果要引用这个信息，一定要阅读原始文献，并直接引用原始文献。只有在特殊情况下引用间接文献，比如原始文献找不到，或者采用为非自己懂得的文字撰写的。在这种情况下，也要指出原始文献。

如作者阅读了 Li 等人（2000）的文章，其中引用了 Huang（1800），但作者自己无法找到 Huang 的作品，则注明 Huang 的作品作为原始来源，但只有 Li 等人的作品出现在参考文献列表中。文章中注明："by Huang（1800），as cited in Li et al.（2000）"。

又如，我们在 Zhao 的文章中提到《黄帝内经》，但我们没有读过，或者读者一般也不会读《黄帝内经》，则可以写："by Inner Canon of Huangdi（as cited in Zhao et al, 2000）"。

第 7 节　引入参考文献的常用词汇

1. 引入历史研究

> It is now well established that…

> Many recent studies have shown that…

> Several lines of evidence suggest that…

> Data from several studies suggest that…

> The literature on X has highlighted several…

> There are relatively few studies in the area of…

> A number of studies have assessed the efficacy of…

> Several studies have used longitudinal data to examine…

> The vast majority of studies on X have been quantitative.

> A large and growing body of literature has investigated…

> There is a large number of published studies that describe…

> What we know about X is largely based on observational studies.

> Previous studies have explored the relationships between X and Y.

> In recent years, there has been an increasing amount of literature on…

> There is a large volume of published studies describing the role of…

> There is a relatively small body of literature that is concerned with…

> Previous research findings into X have been inconsistent and contradictory

> There are a number of large cross-sectional studies which suggest…

> Two cohort study analyses have examined the relationship between…

> A considerable amount of literature has been published on X. These studies…

> Over the past two decades, major advances in molecular biology have allowed…

> Numerous studies have attempted to explain…. For example, Smith et al reported….

> Around the early 2010s, small-scale research and case studies began to emerge linking…

> At least 10（A number of）case-control studies worldwide have examined the relationship between…

> To date（Thus far/Up to now）several studies（a number of studies，a variety of studies）have found（reported/shown that/indicated that/linked X with Y/suggested that/demonstrated that/confirmed the effectiveness of / revealed a correlation between X and Y）.

2. 突出参考文献的时间

> A recent study by X et al involved…

> In XXXX，X et al. demonstrated that…

> In XXXX，a seminal article was published…

> Preliminary work on X was undertaken by X.

> In a follow-up study, Smith *et al.* found that…

> In XXXX，X et al. reported a new procedure to…

> A recent systematic literature review concluded that…

> Thirty years later，X reported three cases of X which…

> In one well-known recent experiment，X were found to be…

> In XXXX，X et al. published a paper in which they described…

> The first systematic study of X was reported by Y *et al.* in 19XX.

> Analysis of the genes involved in X was first carried out by Y *et al.*

3. 引出他人的观点

> According to X（As noted by X），Y is far more cost effective，and therefore…

> X argues（claims/suggests/concludes/points out/proposes）that X is far more cost effective，and therefore better adapted to the developing world.

4. 引出更多资料的

> Similarly，Y found that X…

> X's data support Y's view that…

> In contrast to X，Y argues that…

> Likewise，W holds the view that…

➢ X's work is complemented by Y's study of…

➢ This view is supported by X who found that…

➢ However，X's study of Y found no link between…

➢ Other researchers，however，have found…，for example，…

➢ Conversely，W reported no significant difference in mortality between X and Y.

5. 引出方法

➢ Samples were analysed as previously reported by X et al.

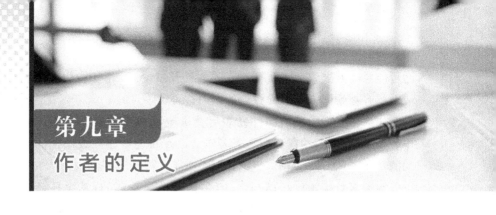

第九章
作者的定义

第 1 节　作者的内涵

科学论文的发表,既是对个人工作的肯定,也涉及个人的职业生涯中的晋升,因此研究者能否成为作者和作者的排名是课题组常常争论的问题。当前杂志基本采用 ICMJE 的作者标准。不符合作者资格的研究者可以在致谢中列出(当然要经过本人同意),最好附有致谢的原因。同样,通常要求作者填写并签署作者确认和利益冲突声明。在大型多中心研究中,可能会选择课题组作为作者,其中主要研究人员被列为主要作者,并注明"on behalf of the XX group",而其他成员在致谢中列出。大多数数据库(如 PubMed)会列出全部作者。

ICMJE 建议作者署名要同时符合以下四条标准:

(1) 对研究概念和设计、数据获取或数据分析和解释做出重大贡献(contributed substantially to the conception and design, acquisition of data, or analysis and interpretation of data)。

(2) 对撰写论文做出重大贡献或对论文的重要知识内容提出关键性的修改建议(contributed to writing the paper or revising it critically for important intellectual content)。

(3) 同意最终的论文版本的发表(given final approval of the version to be published)。

(4) 同意对研究工作的各个方面承担责任,以确保与论文任何部分的准确性或诚信有关的质疑得到恰当的调查和解决。

所有作者都应该满足以上四条标准,而所有满足以上四条标准者也不应该被遗漏。未满足全部四条标准者应该被致谢。致谢可能意味着被致谢人认可研究的数据及结论，因此有些杂志要求通信作者取得所有被致谢人同意被致谢的书面许可。

如果作者在投稿或稿件发表后要求删除或添加某个作者，或变动排名，作者要给出解释，并得到所有署名作者以及将要被删除或添加的作者同意变动的签字声明。一般在审稿结束后杂志不允许作者变动。

在大多数生物医学期刊中，第一作者是最重要的，其次是最后一位作者（Last author，一般是通讯作者 Corresponding author）和第二作者。通常通讯作者一般是第一作者或最后一位作者（也称为 Lead author，Senior author）。大部分期刊允许共同第一作者和共同通讯作者。少部分期刊还要求一位作者作为担保人（Guarantor）。担保人对从研究开始到发表文章的整个研究的完整性负责。在编辑过程中和发表后，通讯作者是论文相关问题的主要联系人。最近也有杂志除了注明谁是"corresponding author"外，还注明谁是"senior author"。

作者的排序既是对其工作应有的肯定，最好在研究项目开始时就要讨论好作者的排序，并签署协议。排序可根据每人完成的工作比例的变化不时进行修改。大多数研究项目将产生多篇论文，每篇论文的作者角色可能不同。在初稿起草之前，负责人要明确谁将担任主要作者。一般来说即使作者改变了工作单位，发表论文的时候标注的单位是论文中的工作实际进行时候所在的单位。

主要作者完成初稿后，每个作者有责任对其完成的部分的数据进行核实，并对文章的撰写提出批判性的意见。投稿前每个作者要仔细检查自己的姓名拼音、头衔和单位。拼错的名字会出现在数据库中，比如 PubMed。

顾名思义，通讯作者是在投稿、同行评议、出版过程中与期刊联系的人，也是出版后和读者交流的主要负责人。将通讯作者作为文章的负责人是一个约定成俗的行规，但随着科学界对通讯作者在行文章中的重要性的默认以及很多单位将通讯作者的重要性视同第一作者，杂志开始对通讯作者提出很高的要求，这是责任和荣誉的统一。这些责任包括：

• 确保作者名单包括了所有应该列入的研究人员，而且顺序、贡献声明已经得到所有作者的同意，投稿时已经通知了所有作者。

• 作为联络人，将出版过程的任何问题告知全部作者。虽然通信作者主要负责与期刊的联系，但很多杂志编辑会将所有的通信发送给全部署名作者。

• 有些杂志只要求通讯作者投稿时候签字。这时通讯作者负责确保所有作者均同意被列为作者，并已同意向期刊投稿。通讯作者还负责代表论文所有作者提交利益冲突声明。

· 确保数据、材料和代码符合期刊的公开(透明性)要求。

· 确保稿件中涉及的原始数据、材料、代码保存完好,以便将来重新分析。

· 保证引用的任何未出版材料(例如个人通信、还没有投稿或正在审稿中的论文)获得了作者的书面许可。保证来自其他地方发表的任何材料(如图)获得了作者和/或出版商的书面许可。

· 作为已发表论文的联系人,有责任将与已发表论文有关的任何事项通知所有作者,并确保这些事项得到及时处理。

· 论文投稿后对作者的任何更改,如更改作者顺序或删除或添加作者,必须得到每位作者的同意。

· 文章发表后一旦受到质疑,期刊会要求提供原始资料或其他信息,通信作者要积极配合。

在 2007 年《自然》的一篇社论中曾经就要求资深作者或通讯作者签署一份声明,声明他们在投稿之前已经采取"诚信保险"步骤,保证文章数据的真实性[1]。结果一些人赞成,但大多数人不赞成。反对的人认为目前科研合作往往是多团队的,要求通讯作者承担此类责任实际上做不到,这种签署的声明最终会流于形式。因此《自然》杂志要求在论文中每个合作小组必须至少有一名成员作为主要作者对其小组的工作负责。主要责任有 3 个:①保存论文所依据的原始数据;②验证数据和结论是否准确反映收集的数据,以及图像处理是否符合杂志指南;③最大限度地减少材料、数据和算法共享的障碍。

联合作者(Consortia authorship)是指一组作者。一般在文章作者中只列出主要作者名单和联合作者的名称,联合作者的成员名单在附件中列出。

为了确保相同名字的作者不会被混淆,越来越多的杂志要求作者必须提供其开放研究者和贡献者标识符(Open Researcher and Contributor Identifier, ORCID)。

第 2 节　作者的贡献

要求作者披露在研究中的贡献(contribution)是因为在历史上发生的多个造假事件的调查过程中，文章中有些作者提出自己并不知道被列入到了作者名单中。确实，有时候有些作者会将一些知名科学家列入名单中，以提高文章被接受的机会。还有就是没有做贡献的人自己提出的要求，也就是所谓的"honorary author(an author unacceptably included for reasons other than any scientific contribution)"。《自然》杂志 1999 年首次出台了作者贡献声明的政策[2]。

作者的贡献可以用 CRediT(Contributor Roles Taxonomy)来描述，一共14 类，但也可以包括其他类别。该分类法已由 Consortia Advancing Standards in Research Administration（CASRAI）和美国 National Information Standards Organization(NISO)改进，被 Cell Press、PLOS 和许多出版商采用。一个人可以有多种贡献，一个任务（贡献）可以有多个人完成。可以采用"lead""equal"和"supporting"来描述贡献的程度。通讯作者负责确认每个人的贡献。每个分类的具体解析如下：

1. 提出概念(Conceptualization)：通常说的 Idea，制定或完善总体研究目标和目的。

2. 数据整理(Data curation)：注释（生成元数据）、清理和维护研究数据（包括解释数据本身所需的软件代码）的管理活动，以供初始使用和以后使用。

3. 正式分析(Formal analysis)：应用统计、数学、计算或其他技术分析或合成研究数据。

4. 资金获取(Funding acquisition)：获取本论文相关研究项目的财务支持。

5. 研究(Investigation)：开展研究，特别是进行实验或数据/证据收集。

6. 方法学(Methodology)：方法的开发或设计，创建模型。

7. 项目管理(Project administration)：负责研究活动的规划和执行方面的管理和协调。

8. 资源(Resources)：提供研究材料、试剂、患者数据、实验室样本、动物、仪器、计算资源或其他分析工具。

9. 软件(Software)：编程、软件开发，计算机程序设计，计算机代码和支持算法的实现；测试现有代码组件。

10. 监管(Supervision)：领导和监督研究活动。

11. 验证(Validation)：对结果/实验和其他研究成果的部分或整体复制和再现。

12. 可视化(Visualization)：准备、创建和/或展示论文的工作，特别是可视化/数据展示。

13. 写作(草稿撰写)(Writing-original draft)：准备、创作和/或展示论文中的工作，特别是撰写初稿(包括主要的翻译)。

14. 写作(评论和编辑)(Writing-review and editing)：批评性审核、评论或修订，包括文章出版前或出版后。

参考文献

[1] Who is accountable？[J]. Nature，2007，450(7166)：1.

[2] Policy on papers' contributors[J]. Nature，1999 3，399(6735)：393.

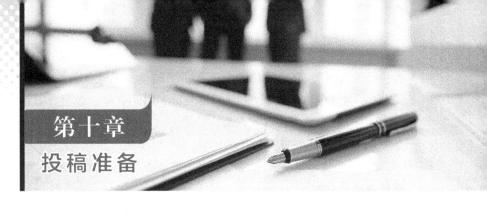

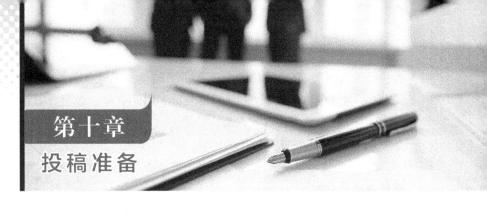

第十章

投稿准备

投稿之前作者应确保以下内容：所述科学问题的清晰性、论文结构的合规性、方法的适当性、所提供数据的正确性、结果解释的合理性、讨论的相关性以及结论的正确性。故事情节是否显而易见、合乎逻辑？语言是否清晰且简洁？术语是否正确？是否有拼写错误（Typo）？如果作者中没有精通英文的，最好请母语人士或专业语言编辑服务机构检查您的论文。

ICMJE 有对论文的统一投稿要求。但每种期刊对论文都有自己的具体要求，如字数、参考文献格式、表格和图表是嵌入（Embedded）论文中还是单独提交等。

第 1 节　期刊选择

为发表论文选择合适的期刊并不容易。通常我们要考虑的主要因素有：

• 读者群：既然写一篇科学论文和讲一个故事是类似的，那么对谁讲呢？显然，你的读者在很大程度上取决于你发表作品的期刊，因为每个期刊都有相对固定的读者群。

• 录用率：根据期刊的知名度、空间限制和投稿量，投稿录用率从最著名期刊的 10% 以下到某些期刊的 80% 以上不等。而没有容量限制的电子期刊的数量不断增加。这类期刊不受篇幅限制，通常每年能够发表更多的论文，并且在论文被接受后很快就能发表。发文量每年以万为单位的期刊被称为 Mega Journal。

• 版面费：现在许多科学期刊采用全部或部分开放存取（Open access，OA）。不订阅该杂志的人也可以阅读论文（例如低收入国家的研究人员）。OA 期刊一般收取 5 000～20 000 元人民币的出版费,取代了传统的读者付费的商业模式。经典的杂志可以选择OA和不付费的方式出版,但录用率较低。因此要考虑版面费的预算有多少。

此外,还需要考虑以下方面:

1. 指导老师或资深同行的经验。

2. 看看自己论文的参考文献发表的杂志,或通过检索看看类似的研究在哪些杂志发表过。

3. 你是更在乎杂志的读者群,还是更在乎能够快速发表? 投经典的专业杂志可能会有更多的同行阅读您的文章,但竞争可能很大。

4. 杂志的文章偏向基础研究还是临床研究? 是全科杂志还是专科杂志? 是传统的(印刷)期刊还是电子期刊?

5. 制定一份3~5个期刊的优先列表。当被拒稿的时候可以节约再次投稿的时间。

6. 影响因子虽然是一个备受争议但仍被广泛使用的衡量期刊在该领域相对重要性的指标,也是投稿人重要的选刊指标。期刊的影响因子反映了过去两年期刊上发表文章的平均引用次数。

7. 看看期刊的网站和投稿说明;仔细阅读目录和论文,了解期刊的范围和编辑的偏好。

8. 了解杂志的论文审稿和出版周期,平衡好在高影响因子期刊上发表的可能性和希望发表的时间。向拒稿率高的期刊提交论文可能会给您提供有价值的审稿意见,但也可能会因为需要多次投稿而延长出版过程。此外,这些高端杂志可能没有审稿就直接被拒稿了。

9. 搜索相关杂志是最近否有特刊(Special issues)和论文征集(Calls for papers),看看是否正好符合您的研究内容。

10. 采用辅助工具寻找目标杂志。如Journal Suggester,Journal Finder,可以输入摘要后获得提示[1,2]。

切记,一次只能将论文投一个期刊。

第 2 节　开放存取出版方式

OA 是互联网时代下催生的出版方式,适用于杂志和电子书。在这种方式下读者可以通过知识共享许可(Creative Commons License)在文章出版后立即免费获取文章,并且通常没有或很少有使用的限制。OA 方式下作者保留作品的版权。杂志出版社的运营依靠投稿人支付的出版费(Article publishing charge,APC)。国际上 AOC 从 600 美元到 3 000 美元不等,和杂志的影响度相关。通常没有被 SCI 收录的杂志不收 APC。

相比之下,当论文在传统订阅方式的期刊上(Subscription journal)发表时,不用支付 APC,但需要把论文的版权转让给出版社,出版社拥有版权。读者需要向出版社付费后才能订阅或下载论文。杂志出版社的运营依靠读者、机构用户、个人用户的付费和广告收入。

有两种 OA 类型。"金 OA"意味着读者可以在文章发布后立即自由阅读和下载文章。"绿色 OA"适用于订阅模式下发表的文章。一定时间后(通常为12 个月)文章可以在任何非营利性网站公开。这个时间段称为"embargo period"。"绿色 OA"模式下杂志社通常拥有该论文的版权。期刊可以采用"金 OA""绿色 OA"或混合出版模式。投稿到混合模式期刊时作者可自由选择付费+保留版权的模式和不付费+版权转让的模式。细胞出版社(Cell Press)把"绿色 OA"称为开放存档(open archive)。

有些投稿人认为花钱选择 OA 模式会促进混合出版的杂志社接受投稿,这是误解,因为一般杂志在论文接受后才要求投稿人选择出版方式。

第 3 节　期刊指标

期刊指标(Journal metrics)是衡量一个杂志的定量工具,可以帮助你选择期刊。然而每个指标都有其局限性,只反映了期刊质量和影响力的一部分,因此不应单独考虑。常用的期刊指标包括:

使用率(Usage):Online 用户在上一年阅读该杂志文章的总次数。

影响因子(Impact factor):在两年的时间窗口内,期刊上发表的文章的平均被引用数。只有 Clarivate 科学引文索引(Science Citation Index Expanded,

SCIE)或社会科学引文索引(Social Sciences Citation Index，SSCI)中的期刊具有影响因子。

影响因子最佳四分位数(Best quartile)：期刊在引用报告中的相关主题类别排名。Q1＝影响因子排名前 25％ 的期刊。

5 年影响系数：五年内期刊文章的平均引用次数。

CiteScore(Scopus)：四年内该杂志文章收到的平均引用次数。

CiteScore 最佳四分位数：该杂志在 Scopus 学科类别中的 CiteScore 排名。Q1 的期刊处于最高的核心位置。

SJR(Scimago Journal Rank)：一年内的平均(加权)引用数除以前三年在该杂志上发表的文章数。

从提交到第一个决定的时间：上一年提交给期刊的稿件收到第一个决定的平均或中位数天数。有些期刊的这个时间的中位数为"0 天"，这是什么原因？因为一些期刊在收到的论文中有很大一部分被拒绝，而没有将其发送给同行评审(即所谓的 Desk rejection)。如果这类期刊的效率很高，通常在论文提交的同一天做出是否拒稿的决定，那么平均速度可能不到一天。从提交到第一次收到审稿回复的时间是一个有用的指标，它表明如果你的文章被选中进行同行审核，你可能需要多长时间才能收到审稿决定。

从提交到第一次收到审稿回复的时间：如果稿件发送给同行评审，提交给期刊的稿件收到第一次审稿意见的平均或中位数天数。这也是上年的数据。

从稿件被接受到在线发布的时间：这也是上年的数据，为平均或中位数天数。

稿件接受率：上年发表的文章占收到所有投稿论文的百分比。

为什么没有一个从投稿到文章出版的速度指标？速度指标的目的是让期刊编辑、审稿和出版商能够控制或影响的时间变得透明。然而从投稿到文章出版的时间还包括作者回复审稿意见的时间，而这个时间不同的作者差异很大，和杂志无关，因此期刊的指标不包含这个。比如，《Lancet》曾经对重要的 RCT 研究(Practice-changing trials)推出了 10＋10 政策，即 10 天的审稿时间和 10 天的作者回复到 online 时间，但并不强制要求作者在 10 天内完成回复(Authors can opt for a more leisurely pace if they prefer)[3]。

几乎所有期刊都采用在线投稿系统提交论文。通常 1～2 小时左右可以完成。如果不能一次性完成，系统通常允许保存信息并在以后继续。要警惕采用电子邮件投稿的杂志可能是假冒的杂志。

第 4 节　Cover Letter

Cover Letter 是随论文提交的,一般编辑通过 Cover Letter 开始了解您的研究。因此,Cover Letter 要强调论文对研究领域的意义以及与目标期刊的相关性。Cover Letter 要明确说明作者遵守了杂志的投稿要求,一定要包含编辑可能感兴趣的信息。

大多数期刊希望作者推荐两到三位审稿人,他们是论文相关领域的专家,能够对论文进行客观的评估。期刊可能会联系这些人。有些期刊还要求作者指出不希望作为审稿人的同行专家(如作者和他们在学术上有不同意见)。

Cover Letter 是向编辑"推销你的论文"的很好机会。Cover Letter 应包括以下基本要素:

(1) 希望提交的论文在期刊上发表。

(2) 总结论文的意义(用 2～3 句话):它解决了哪些相关问题,主要发现,以及为什么这一发现很重要。

(3) 指出该论文适合目标杂志的读者的原因。一个很好的理由是相关的工作早些时候发表在目标杂志上。确保你引用了这篇文章,因为这表明了你对该杂志的了解和兴趣。

(4) 没有同时在其他杂志投稿的声明。

(5) 利益冲突的声明。

完成提交后,杂志会将稿件编号发送到通讯作者的邮箱。定期登录投稿系统查看稿件的状态,如果状态不清楚或很长时间没有进展(如 3 个月内一直显示处于"in review"的状态)可以在投稿系统联系编辑询问。

第 5 节　最后的修改

投稿前每个作者在阅读草稿后都尽量提意见,包括内容和写作上的意见,使论文经过 5～10 次的修改后达到精品的水准。最后定稿的时候可以尝试大声阅读稿件,以了解句子的通顺程度和组织水平。重点检查以下内容:

- 有没有重复的内容。

- 检查表格和图的内容是否正确:缩写、单位、统计学符号。

- 检查表格和图的标题和说明是否清晰和简洁。
- 阅读杂志的作者须知,核对稿件是否符合。

参考文献

[1] https://authorservices. taylorandfrancis. com/publishing-your-research/choosing-a-journal/journal-suggester.

[2] https://journalfinder. elsevier. com.

[3] The Lancet. 10+10: rapid decisions and fast track publication for RCTs[J]. Lancet, 2015;385(9968):578.

I keep six honest serving-men (They taught me all I knew). Their names are What and Why and When and How and Where and Who.

—Rudyard Kipling(1865—1936). *The Elephant's Child*

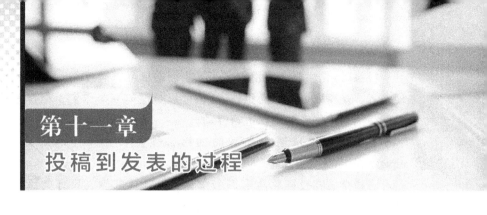

第十一章

投稿到发表的过程

　　作者在投稿之前应考虑论文的主题是否符合期刊的使命（Mission or scope）。如有疑问，作者可向编辑发送电子邮件进行咨询。在决定提交后，在 Cover Letter 中，解释为什么论文适合该杂志。同样重要的是强调该研究相对已有研究的价值。如果该杂志在最近有发表过相同主题的论文，则可以提出，并进行对照，以显示本研究的新发现。

第 1 节　投稿

　　在电脑和互联网时代之前，作者将打字机打印的稿件、手工画图（如线图）和照片一起邮寄到杂志社。此后出现了采用光盘刻录后邮寄给编辑部的方法和电子邮件发送的方法。到了 2000 年左右出现了专业的稿件处理软件，集成了网络投稿、审稿、编辑部管理和出版社管理的功能，如《Vascular Investigation and Therapy》杂志的投稿界面（图 11.1）：

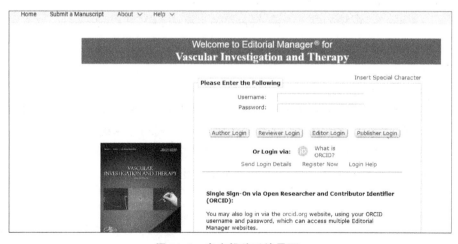

图 11.1　杂志投稿系统界面

投稿时,先注册一个用户名。有些杂志也可以通过 ORCID 账号登录,方便作者。投稿人可以是通讯作者,也可以是任何一个作者。但有些杂志要求只能使用通讯作者的邮箱进行互动。

有些杂志要求通讯作者的邮箱必须是研究机构的邮箱(Academic email),不接受商业邮箱(如 G-mail)。

有些杂志在投稿后会给每个作者发送确认邮件。只有全部作者确认后才会进入审稿流程,因此如果有些作者平时很少看邮件,投稿人要通知每个作者注意查收并确认。如:

Co-author manuscript submission confirmation

Manuscript:EJDERM-2023-47-(161)-Successful therapy of pityriasis lichenoideset varioliformis acuta with dupilumab.

Authors:XXX(Co-author),ZZZ(Co-author),YYY(Corresponding author)

Date submitted:2023-02-22

Dear Dr. XXX

Automatic notification:

The above manuscript has been submitted online by Miss YYY and you have been listed as a co-author.

Please use the link below to:

1. Confirm you are a co-author

2. Confirm that you have given Miss YYY permission to act on your behalf concerning this manuscript submission.

CONFIRM YOU ARE A CO-AUTHOR

If you are NOT a co-author,please contact the editorial office immediately by replying to this email …

Sincerely,

The Editorial Office

必须遵守字数限制。有些数据和表格可以补充材料,以便有兴趣的读者可以看到,如作者设计的调查问卷、详细的数学公式和计算机编程等。

提交时,作者必须写明任何潜在的利益冲突和所有财务支持来源。

作者建议的审稿人不能是直接的同事或最近的合作者。

第 2 节　稿件的一般处理程序

为了不浪费作者不必要的等待时间,对明显不可能接受的投稿,编辑会立刻做出拒稿的决定,方便作者加快向其他杂志投稿。编辑有责任不要浪费总是忙碌的审稿人的宝贵时间。此外,编辑有责任为他们的杂志选择真正好的论文。因此收到稿件时编辑首先会评估稿件是否适合该杂志。以下情况下将立刻予以拒稿:

- 稿件的主题明显不在《Information for authors》中所述的专业范围内。

- 稿件存在无法弥补的明显缺陷(例如,缺少合理的研究目标或研究问题,或文章结构不符合要求,或写作非常糟糕)。

- 编辑认为论文存在明显的利益冲突,仅仅披露也无法解决。在这种情况下,可以咨询编辑的意见。

总而言之,未经审稿直接被拒是相当常见的。

如果提交的稿件已通过编辑评估,则杂志通常会邀请两名审稿人。审稿人必须具有专业知识,是有经验的研究者,并且应该披露与提交的论文或其作者有关的任何可能的利益冲突。

审稿人将评估论文的科学性。他们会尽可能提出具有建设性的修改建议,建议编辑接受或拒绝论文。审稿人可以匿名,也可以公开身份。

在收到审稿意见后,编辑将权衡这些意见后决定直接接受、拒稿或要请作者修改后再投稿。这个过程可能会重复多次。编辑也会从自己的角度添加评论。当审稿人之间的意见差异很大时,编辑可以亲自审稿后做出决定。有时可能会选择邀请第三位审稿人,并根据其意见做出终审。

当作者决定接受修稿的邀请时要在修改稿中对审稿人和编辑提出的所有观点逐一回答。如果作者不同意审稿人的意见,则应在重新提交的信函中明确说明原因。

对于重新提交的稿件,编辑一般会邀请审稿人再次审稿。也有可能权衡这些回复后决定拒稿。一般来说修订次数不超过两次,以避免浪费作者和审稿人的时间。

第3节　同行评议

同行评议(Peer review)指由编辑部之外的专家对投给期刊的稿件进行批评性的评价。采用编辑部自己的编辑对投稿进行审稿的方法称为"in-house review"。同行评议是提高论文质量的重要措施,也是杂志被 SCI 收录的基本要求。同行评议能帮助作者和编辑改进论文的质量。

杂志要及时邀请到足够数量(至少两个)高质量的审稿人是很不容易的。审稿人的意见包含对作者的意见(通常匿名)和给编辑的意见。给编辑的意见不会转发给作者。审稿人对文章的评论和对是否接受的意见常常彼此不同。

主编或相关专业的副主编会充分考虑审稿人的意见,无论是正面的还是负面的,并结合审稿人的意见和自己的判断做出决定。如果编辑发现研究工作存在诚信问题,可在发表前的任何时间拒稿,包括录用后。

每种期刊为每一篇稿件选择审稿人的数量,审稿过程是否为盲审,以及审稿内容是否公开都有所不同。

有些期刊编辑要求在接受论文发表之前有独立的生物统计学家对临床试验数据进行统计分析,有些则要求作者说明研究数据是否可供第三方查看、使用和再分析,还有一些则鼓励或要求作者与他人共享他们的数据用于回顾和再分析。

期刊的投稿是保密的,过早泄露稿件的任何或全部细节都可能损害作者的利益。因此审稿人应该对稿件及其中包含的信息严格保密。在稿件发表之前,审稿人不得公开讨论作者的研究工作,不得盗用作者的思想。审稿人不得将稿件留作私用,在提交审稿意见之后应当销毁稿件副本。

审稿人如果存在冲突,应该主动回避,不参与同行评议。

投稿人如果发现稿件信息被泄露可以向杂志社申诉。

收到拒搞的邮件时不要惊慌!许多已发表的论文在被接受之前已被拒绝或修改多次。毕竟审稿人可能为你免费进行了审稿,提出了改进论文的建议。仔细思考一下被拒绝的原因,进一步完善论文,然后向其他杂志投稿。

第 4 节　回复审稿人

论文投稿后收到修改后再投的邀请是件让人高兴的事,说明期刊对你的稿件感兴趣,也意味着如果你对审稿人的评论做出满意的回应,稿件就很有可能被接受。

提交给采用同行评议的期刊的稿件不需要修改直接被接受,是非常少的。

稿件修订是出版过程中的一个关键步骤,因为它可以极大地提高论文的质量。因此作者需要做好充分准备,认真处理编辑和审稿人的意见。

审稿意见分为主要评论(Major comments)和次要评论(Minor comments)。每一条评论包括关于论文特定部分的明确意见,有时还包括修订建议。

修改的决定可分为两类:小修和大修(Minor and major revisions),不同期刊使用的具体术语可能不同,也可能不作区分。小修改意味着审稿人认为稿件适合出版,只要求进行少量修改,例如增加一些数据,进行更深入的讨论、删除多余的材料、更改格式,以及编辑语言。这些通常不是重大问题。大修的原因多种多样,包括论文不同部分之间的不一致、错误的推断、错误的统计分析、不相关的解释,以及假设、研究设计和结论之间的关系。可能需要作者增加实验、重新分析数据并重写。大修的稿件最后有可能被拒稿。

当收到"修改并重新提交"的决定时,仔细阅读和理解审稿人的意见进行修改并回复。除了简要回复审稿人的意见外,说明在论文中的何处进行了修改。以现在时态或完成时表示对论文的修订,例如,"We now present data on […] in Table 1."; "We have added information on […]"。在修订后的论文中使用文字处理器的"跟踪更改(Track changes)"标记更改的文本。

无论是大修还是小修都需要认真对待,只有审稿人的所有疑问和建议都得到满意的解决,稿件才可能被接受。虽然有时候大修是一个非常累人和棘手的过程,有些作者甚至选择改投其他期刊,但建议还是尽量不要改投。

修订尽量早完成,尤其是在小修的情况下,这样论文在评稿人的脑海中仍然是新鲜的,这可加速评审。延迟到最后一分钟交可能会给编辑和审稿人一个潜在的错误印象,即该研究不是作者的优先事项,或者存在难以解决的严重问题。这会降低他们对作者论文的热情和兴趣,并可能导致不良后果。当然在需要重大修订情况下,作者应仔细利用允许的时间,确保全面理解审稿人的意见,并仔细修改然后回复。

在回复时遵循"三条黄金法则":完整、礼貌和有证据。

作者有责任回答编辑和审稿人提出的所有问题，无论是次要问题还是主要问题。此外作者应在写给编辑的信中明确说明修改了哪些部分，以便编辑和审稿人在对修订稿进行再审时可以快速找到修改的内容，节省时间和精力。

不建议作者批评审稿人的评论或与他们争论。作者应记住，修改稿将被送回同一位审稿人，因此要礼貌且冷静地书写。如一般这样说："Although we understand the concern raised by the reviewer, we disagree because of…"，而不是仅仅说："We disagree."

所有回复均应基于证据，包括相关文献和自己的数据。在作者不同意审稿人意见的情况下，这一点尤为重要。当作者觉得某些评论不准确或源于对其研究的误解时，可以反驳这些观点。在这种情况下作者应该提供证据支持，包括引用你自己的数据或以前发表的论文的证据，清楚地陈述不同意的原因。

你可能会看到两位审稿人相互矛盾的意见。如果发生这种情况要清楚地表达您的立场，并在回复时提及相互矛盾的意见。如果矛盾非常严重，请毫不犹豫地联系编辑。此外，可能会有超出您能力范围的意见。例如，可能会要求你提供病理学证据，或提供不可能的随访信息。在这些情况下，向审稿人承认做不到并解释原因通常可以获得认可。

在回复审稿人的评论时要始终尊重他们。向每位审稿人致谢，感谢他们花时间提出改进建议，并尽可能按照他们的建议修改。当然也可以不同意审稿人的评论。在任何情况下，阅读您的回复和修改后的论文的审稿人都应该得到这样的印象：你认真对待了他们的评论，并且你已经尽了最大努力来改进论文。最后，你会在你的邮箱中找到那封被寄予厚望的电子邮件，标题是"接受出版（Accepted for publication）"。

附 回信模板

＜杂志名字＞

＜论文题目和稿号＞

Dear Editor,

Thank you for your useful comments and suggestions on the language and structure of our manuscript.

We have modified the manuscript accordingly, and detailed corrections are listed below point by point.

1.

2.

3.

4.

The manuscript has been resubmitted to your journal. We look forward to your positive response.

Sincerely,

<通讯作者签名>

PS. Response to revierers'comments

1) In its current state, the level of English throughout your manuscript does not meet the journal's required standard.

A:We have revised the WHOLE manuscript carefully and tried to avoid any grammar or syntax errors. In addition, we have asked several colleagues who are skilled authors of English language papers to check the manuscript. We believe that the language is now acceptable for the review process.

2) Please note that your abstract has exceeded the maximum length of 150 words.

A: The abstract has been revised and its word count is now 149.

3) In your manuscript，Fig. 6 is provided but not cited.

Q: Now all figures are provided and cited in sequence in the main text.

4) A cover letter should include the following statement：… This is not seen in your cover letter.

A: The required information is now included in the cover letter.

5) Please note that the reference style must conform strictly to the journal's Guide for Authors.

A: We have checked all the references and formatted them strictly according to the Guide

第5节　校　对

接受的论文经过排版后杂志社会要求作者进行校对。校对常常用表格的方式(Author Query Form)进行,如:

Dear Author，

It is recommended that you check your typeset manuscript carefully，as some sections may have incurred extensive edits. Also，some queries may have arisen，or some suggestions may be made，which will be listed below. Please check your typeset proof carefully and mark any corrections in the margin of the proof or compile them as a separate list.

Journal of Perinatal Medicine trusts you find these comments and suggestions helpful. However，we wish to emphasise that the responsibility for the content of the manuscript remains entirely with the author(s).

Queries and/or suggestions

Manuscript page/ section/line	Queries/comments	Author's response
JPM 2009049	'Left' 'Right' and 'Middle' in text referring to figures have been changed to 'A' 'B' and 'C'. Please check and confirm if correct.	We have checked and confirm it is correct.
	Reference 16 is not cited in text.	We cited it in the revised manuscript.
Materials and methods	Please explain EDTA.	EDTA＝ethylenediaminetetraacetic acid

有些出版社要求在 PDF 上修改。有些则要求对需要修改的地方以文字说明的方法描述。

在投稿过程中会碰到的词汇：

"Manuscript"：投稿，稿件。提交时的格式通常为 Word 或 LaTeX 文档。

"Copyediting"：文案编辑。对投稿的语法、拼写进行检查，修改文字，提高可读性。

"Typesetting"：排版。将投稿转换成杂志的文章格式的过程。

"Proof"：校样。接受的投稿排版完成后出版社将发给作者进行检查。同时出版社会将他们做的修改或发现的问题告诉作者，要求作者确认。作者要进行仔细的检查，尤其是作者单位和姓名。

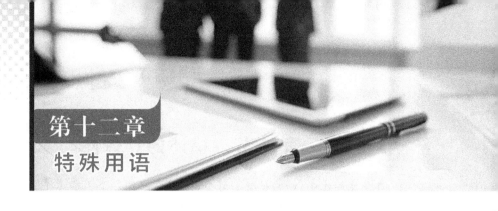

第十二章　特殊用语

医学用词和公共语言是有区别的,作者要留意自己专业的特殊用语。

第1节　研究对象的描述

医学研究对象通用的词包括"patients""participants"和"subjects"。也可以用具体的词来描述研究对象,如"college students""children"和"respondents"。

也有杂志建议不用"subjects",认为不够尊重研究对象,但在统计学中的固定用法除外,如"within-subjects design"和"between-subjects design"。

通常当研究对象接受因为身体或精神问题而接受治疗时,我们可以称他们为"patients"。如果研究的场地不是在医院,而是在学校、公司等的时候,用"patients"则不合适。

"Case"和"person(patient)"有不同的含义。"Case"强调疾病,"person(patient)"强调患病的人。如"manic-depressive cases were treated"应该用"the patients with bipolar disorder were treated"。

第2节　第一人称可以用吗?

虽然有人推崇没有第一人称(No first-person)的习惯,即作者不能在论文中使用"I"或"we",必须用第三人称来称呼自己。例如,"the author"或"the authors",但实际上医学杂志鼓励使用第一人称,以避免歧义!例如,使用"we interviewed participants"而不是"the authors interviewed participants"。其他如:

"We think…";"We believe…";"We concluded…";"Our results showed…"

第3节　描述的具体性

在学术写作中,精确是必不可少的;当你提到一个人或多个人时,选择准确、清晰的词语。例如,用"man"来指代所有人就不如用"individuals""people"或"persons"这样准确。

此外,文章只需要描述和研究相关的特征。虽然可以在文章中包含一个人的年龄、残疾程度、性取向、民族、社会经济地位等特征,但如果这些信息和研究的指标无关,则不需要包含这些信息。例如,在评价药物的抗肿瘤研究中一般不必包括社会经济地位。

对于描述的特征,选择适当具体的术语,方便读者理解,方便其他研究人员在做荟萃分析的时候使用你的数据。

写年龄时,确切的年龄或年龄范围(如 10～15 岁、60～80 岁)比广泛的类别(如 15 岁以下、60 岁以上)更具体。

在写关于残疾的文章时,疾病名称(如 Alzheimer's disease)比疾病类别(如 dementia)更具体。

在写参与研究的人时,"patients""participants""clients"比一般术语(如 people、women)更具体。

在写关于性取向的文章时,取向名称(如 lesbians、gay men、bisexual people、straight people)比广义群体标签(如 gay)更具体。

在写社会经济地位时,收入范围(如 below the state poverty threshold for a family of four)比一般标签(如 low income)更具体。

尽量不要用组的缩写,如不要用"LV group"代替 the low verbal group。采用 Group A、B、C 的方法虽然可以,但读者阅读起来很费力。

第4节　注意敏感性词汇

避免敏感词汇,确保人们的个性和人性得到尊重。避免使用形容词作为名词来标记人(例如,the gays, the poor)或用疾病名称描述病人(例如,amnesiacs,健忘症患者;schizophrenics,精神分裂症患者;the learning disabled,学习障碍者;drug users,吸毒者)。可以使用形容词短语形式(例如,

gay men, older adults)或带有描述性短语的名词（例如，people living in poverty, people with learning disabilities, people who use drugs）。

比较群体要谨慎。一般不要使用"normal group"这样的词汇，这样可能会促使读者将其他组归为"异常"，从而使其他组的个体因差异而蒙受耻辱。同样，将女同性恋者与"normal women"进行对比，会暗示女同性恋处于社会边缘。

社会群体呈现的顺序可能会让读者误会为作者认为第一个提到的群体是规范或标准的，而后面提到的群体是不正常的。因此，"men and women"和"White Americans and racial minorities"这两个短语微妙地反映了在谈论种族和民族身份时，男性和白人相对重要地位。同样，在呈现群体数据时，将男性和白人等社会群体放在图表左侧或表格顶部也可能意味着这些群体是普遍标准。因此为了避免此类情况发生，当提到多个群体时，可以采用字母顺序或样本大小顺序等方法排列。而且在一篇论文中始终以相同的顺序列出各组。

第 5 节　Person-first 和 Identity-first

残疾(Disability)是一个宽泛的术语，包括身体、心理、智力和社会情感障碍，从法律和科学的角度有不同的内含。某些残疾人群体有自己的特殊称呼方式，他们希望其他人采用这种称呼方式，我们要尊重他们的偏好，要了解 Person-first 和 Identity-first 两种语言习惯。

很多人推崇 Person-first 用法，这样可以避免在一个人前面贴上一个疾病的标签。Person-first 用法的例子：

> person with a disability
> patient with cancer
> people with dwarfism
> child who has cerebral palsy
> person with AIDS
> individuals with disabilities。

推广 person-first 语言可以追溯到 20 世纪 60 年代末开始的 People First 运动。person-first 语言在 20 世纪 90 年代变得更加普遍。1990 年《美国残疾人法案》将 person-first 语言确立为许多政府文件和媒体中的首选措辞。

Person-first 语言在很大程度上已经成为医学领域的首选方法。世界卫生组织（World Health Organization）和美国疾病控制与预防中心（US Centers for Disease Control and Prevention）等主要卫生组织，以及美国医学会（American Medical Association）和心理学会（American Psychological Association）的指南都采用 Person-first 语言。

而推崇 Identity-first 的人则认为这样可以强调个人的特征，因为这个特征非常重要。例如："autistic person"，"blind child"。很多病人群体推崇使用 Identity-first（如 blind，deaf，autistic people）。但这些病人群体内部其实也是有分歧的。

适合用：person with paraplegia，person with quadriplegia，person with an intellectual disability，person with a cognitive disability.

不适合用：paraplegic person，quadriplegic person，intellectually disabled person，cognitively disabled person.

自闭症：尽管一些倡导组织历史上推荐使用 Person-first 语言（如 a person with autism；an adult on the autism spectrum），但对 Identity-first 语言的偏好日益增长。许多盲人、聋人和自闭症社区的成员现在更提倡 Identity-first，他们认为这种特征是他们身份的一个组成部分，应该自豪地强调，而不是让他们感到羞耻或需要"治愈"的东西。

耳聋：Identity-first 语言也在很大程度上被聋人群体所接受（当提到与聋人文化相关的事物时，通常用大写的 Deaf）。许多主要组织，如美国聋人协会和世界聋人联合会，都提倡 Identity-first 语言，如"deaf person""deaf Americans"和"Deaf community"。尽管如此，有些人还是喜欢 Person-first 语言（如 a person who is deaf）。

不用：person with deafness，person who is deaf，hearing-impaired person，person who is hearing impaired，person with hearing loss 和 person with deafness and blindness.

可用：Deaf person，hard-of-hearing person，person who is hard-of-hearing 和 Deaf-Blind person.

失明：尽管偏好各不相同，但盲人群体中的个人和组织，包括美国盲人联合会、皇家盲人研究所，以及各个盲人和视力障碍委员会，都普遍偏好并推广 identity-first 语言。

不用：visually challenged person，sight-challenged person，person with blindness，a person who is blind.

可用：blind person，visually impaired person，vision-impaired person，person who is blind，person who is visually impaired 和 person who is vision impaired.

侏儒症和身材矮小：侏儒症患者组织通常同时使用 Person-first 和 Identity-first 语言。当然，个人之间的偏好可能会有所不同。

Person-first 例子：a person who has dwarfism，people of short stature.

Identity-first 例子：dwarf，little person.

对于药物和物质成瘾：人们普遍倾向于使用 Person-first 语言，取代诸如瘾君子（Addict）和酒鬼（Alcoholic）之类的污名化词汇：

➢ a person with alcohol use disorder，people with substance use disorders.

出于类似的原因，关注自杀预防的组织也普遍使用 Person-first 语言：

➢ a person experiencing thoughts of suicide，people impacted by suicide.

如果你不知道或无法确定某个群体使用哪种语言，推荐使用 person-first 语言。但无论如何，尊重该群体的偏好是研究者的专业素养。了解研究对象偏好的最好方法是到他们的群体的官网上看看他们用那种方法。

第6节　消极和屈尊的术语

避免使用暗示限制的或否定性术语以及使用负面标签。

不适合用：AIDS victim，wheelchair bound，confined to a wheelchair 和 brain damaged；

适合用：person with AIDS，wheelchair user 和 person with a traumatic brain injury。

避免使用可能被视为诽谤的术语。

不适合用：cripple（残疾人），nuts（疯子），alcoholic（酒鬼），meth addict（冰毒成瘾者）；

适合用：person with a physical disability，person with a mental illness，person with alcohol use disorder 和 person with substance use disorder。或者更具体一些，例如 person with schizophrenia。

在描述残疾人时，避免使用屈尊的委婉语。

适合用：special needs，physically challenged，mentally challenged，mentally retarded，mentally ill 和 handi-capable。

可用：person with a disability，person who has a disability，disabled person, person with a mental illness, people with intellectual disabilities, child with a congenital disability, child with a birth impairment, physically disabled person 和 person with a physical disability。

第 7 节 年龄用语

"Males""females""person"和"individual"可用于任何年龄的人。

小于等于 12 岁者可用："child"，"girl"和"boy"。

13～17 岁者可用："adolescent"，"young person"，"youth"，"young woman"，"young man"，"female adolescent"和"male adolescent"。

大于等于 18 岁者用："adult"，"woman"，"man"。

老年人尽量注明具体年龄段，否则可用"older persons"，"older people"，"older adults"，"older patients"，"older individuals"和"the older population"。

不用 "seniors"，"elderly"，"the aged"和"senile"。

不用 "the elderly"，"elders"，"elderly people"，"the aged"，"aging dependents"，"seniors"和"senior citizens"。

另外，可以参考 PubMed 的搜索引擎过滤功能中对年龄用语的定义：

Newborn：birth-1 month.

Infant：birth-23 months，或 1～23 months.

Preschool Child：2～5 years.

Child：6～12 years.

Adolescent：13～18 years.

Adult：19～44 years.

Young Adult：19～24 years.

Middle Aged：45～64 years.

Aged：65＋years.

第 8 节 性别用语

"Gender"是指特定文化与一个人的生物性别相关联的态度、情感和行为。"Gender"是一种社会建构和社会认同。当把人们称为社会群体时，使用"gender"一词。例如，作者可用这样写："Approximately 60% of participants identified as cisgender women，35％ as cisgender men，3％ as transgender women，1％ as transgender men，and 1％ as nonbinary. ”

"Sex"指的是生物上的分类（如出生时的性别）。

第 9 节　其　他

不要用"fail"标示否定，因为"fail"强调的是主观意识，而不是结果。因此不要说："Two participants failed to complete the test"，而应该说："… did not complete …"。

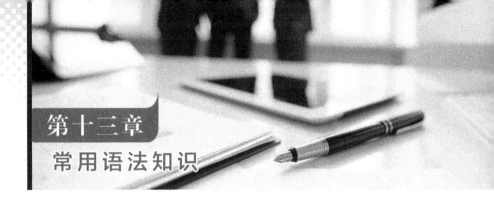

第十三章
常用语法知识

英语的语法主要涉及词类、时态、语态、语气、句型结构和标点符号的使用。

第1节　标点符号

医学论文常用的标点符号包括逗号（Comma）、分号（Semicolon）、冒号（Colon）、句号（Period）、问号（Question mark）、破折号（Dash）、括号（Parentheses）和方括号（Square bracket）。

英文没有顿号，采用逗号取代。逗号、分号、冒号、句号和问号后面要有一个空格（个别杂志要求两个空格）。

标点符号确定句子的节奏，告诉读者在哪里暂停（逗号、分号和冒号）、停止（句号和问号）或改变（破折号、括号和方括号）。

串行逗号（也称为系列逗号）用于由三个或更多项组成的名词或词组之间。如：

➤ Factors of personality include extraversion, conscientiousness, openness to experience, agreeableness, and neuroticism.

如果序列中的一个或多个项目已包含逗号，则在项目之间使用分号，而不是逗号。如：

➤ Subjective well-being is characterized by the presence of positive affect, such as happy feel; the absence of negative affect, such as angry feel; and a high level of life satisfaction.

➤ We divided participants by age into categories of young adults, whose ages are between 18 to 40 years; middle-aged adults, whose ages are between 40 and 60 years; and older adults, whose ages are 60 years and older.

有些相隔的词组比较复杂，或者为了突出词组之间的平行关

第十三章　常用语法知识　153

系,可以采用字母序列(Lettered list)。如:Participants provided information about their (a) level of education; (b) incomes; (c) occupation; and (d) marriage status.

编号列表(Numbered list):显示一系列完整的句子或段落(例如,逐项列出的结论、操作步骤)。使用文字处理程序的编号列表功能来创建编号列表。如:

Our hypotheses were as follows:

1. Old patients use more pills.
2. Old patients have more diseases.
3. Old patients visit hospital more often.

第 2 节　列　表

≫ 项目符号列表(Bulleted List)

如果项目的排列不需要特定顺序(例如,时间顺序、重要性、优先级),可使用项目符号列表。如果项目是完整的句子,则以大写字母开头,以句号或其他适当的标点符号结束。如:

Pertinent were excluded if they met the following criteria:

- They were older than 80 years.
- They were pregnant.
- They had hypertension.

如果项目是单词或短语,每个项目以小写字母开头(专有名词等单词除外)。

当项目为单词或短语时,项目符号列表的标点有两个形式。第一种形式是在项目(包括最后一个项目)后不使用标点符号,适合较短的项目。如:

Hypertension has been linked with the following:

- high BMI
- low physical activity
- stress
- smoking

第二种形式适合长的项目,后面用标点符号。如:

Texts are used for：

- social connection，in which people text as a way to connect with others.

- audacity，in which people text to get a response from someone，such as to break up with them or ask them on a date；and

- nurturing，in which people text to foster relationships by saying things like "good morning" or "I love you".

第3节　医学词汇的连字符使用规则

复合词通常有三种形式：

- 每个单词独立，如：Health care。

- 采用连字符，如：Self-esteem。

- Solid word，如：Caregiver。

医学文献中有较多的临时复合词（Temporary compound word）。临时复合词是指词典中还没有收录的词。临时复合词一般加连字符，以避免误解，如"high-anxiety group"。

前缀后面一般不加连字符，如"antisocial"，"covariate"，"nonsignificant"，"overqualified"，"preexisting"，"prosocial"，"postgraduate"，"reevaluate"，"unbiased"，"underdiagnosis"和"underappreciated"。

第4节　首字母大写

专有名词（Proper noun）一般首字母大写。医学中常用的专有名词是种族和族裔群体的名称，例如："African American"，"Asian American"，"Black"，"European American"，"First Nations"，"Hispanic"，"Native American"，"Latinx"，"White"。

商品名首字母大写（例如，药物的品牌名称）。但是药物的通用名称不大写。

第 5 节　数　字

医学论文中数字是必不可少的,如参与者人数、年龄等人口统计信息以及统计分析结果。

一般而言,0~9 的数字用文字表示,10 以上用阿拉伯数字。如:

➤ There were five patients.

➤ Students were in the third, sixth, eighth, 10th, and the 12th grades.

➤ The study had 40 participants.

但以下情况用文字:

在句子、标题或标题开头的数字(有时候通过改写句子以避免以数字开头):"Fifty percent of the patients received treatment A, and the other 50% received treatment B."

分数:"one fifth of the class; two-thirds majority."

以下情况用数字(表 13.1):

表 13.1　需用数字的情况

情况	举例
计量单位前面	1-mg dose, 3 cm
数学函数	multiplied by 2
分数	1.5
百分比	50%
比例	4 : 1 ratio
百分位(Percentiles),四分位	the 5th percentile, the 95th percentile the 3rd quartile
时间和日期	3 s, 3 min, 3 hr, 3 days, 3 months, 3 years about 3 years ago, 3 decades, 12:30 a.m.
年龄	3 years old, 30 years old 3-year-olds, 30-year-olds 3-year-old children, 30-year-old adults
量表	scored 3 on a 10-point scale
名词后	Step 1, Grade 5, Grade 11, Table 2, and Figure 5

注意:Column 8, Row 7, Chapter 6, Chapter 14 中名词首字母大写,但页和段用缩写和小写:p. 3, pp. 1~3, para. 3, paras. 1~3。

第 6 节 作为单数的"They"

单数"they"是英语中通用的第三人称单数代词,避免对性别做出假设。尽管在学术写作中曾经不鼓励使用单数"they",但许多出版社已经接受并认可了它,包括《韦氏词典》。若果确信描述的对象中有男有女,则可用"he or she"和"she or he",但不要有"(s)he" and "s/he"。

例句如表 13.2:

表 13.2 例句

Form	Example
they	Casey is a gender-fluid person. They are from Texas.
them	Every patient received a care package delivered to them.
their	Each child played with their parent.
theirs	The cup of coffee is theirs.
themselves(or themself)	A private person usually keeps to themselves [or themself].

虽然"they"代表单数,但其后面用复数动词(即用"they are",不用"they is")。

代表单数的时候"themselves"和"themself"都可以。不过"themselves"更加常用。

如果感觉用"they"作为第三人称单数不通顺,可以尝试其他替代的办法,如:"I delivered a care package to the patient"。

第 7 节 缩 写

缩写一般只能用于名词,在第一次出现的时候注明,而且一定要在此后的全文中使用。非名词的临床上常用的缩写,可以用于表格和图,但一般不用于正文中,如"once a day"(不用"qd"),"twice a day"(不用"bid"),"thrice a day"(不用"tid")和"4 times a day"(不用"qid")。

如果在章节标题中首次使用缩写,全称不要在标题中展开,要在该章节的文本中首次使用时展开缩写。

基因名称、限制性内切酶名称、细胞系和小鼠品系只用缩写,不用加全称。其他常用、不加全称说明的词有:AIDS,DNA,HIV,HLA,MAPK,$PaCO_2$,PaO_2,RNA 和 UV 等。

第8节　避免口语和非正式用词

不要使用惯用或口语词汇:不用"kids",用"children"

不要用动词缩略形式"don't"和"can't";用"do not"和"can not".

介绍例子不用"like",用"such as"或"for instance"。

很多不用"lots of",用"a significant/considerable number"。

大小不用"little/big",用"small/large:a small/ large proportion of the patients"。

不用"get"词组,如"get better/worse",用"improve"或"deteriorate"。

效果不用"good/bad",用"positive/negative",如"the changes had several positive aspects"。

写清单时,避免使用"etc"或"so on"。

能够用一个词的单词的时候,不要用两个词的动词:如不用"go on"或"bring up";使用"continue"或"raise"。

下面是其他常用的非正式语,而括号中的是推荐使用的正式语。

a lot of(much, many), do(perform, carry out, conduct), think(consider), talk(discuss), look at(examine), get(obtain), keep(retain, preserve),really 和 things(写具体的对象)。

避免使用主观色彩的词,如"gigantic""beautiful""nice""fantastic"和"enormous"。

第9节　客观原则

科学英语必须客观。一般来说,尽量减少使用人称代词(例如 we,our),因为这些代词会降低科学论文的客观性。因此,"From our analysis, we found that radiation led to cell death."最好改为:"This analysis showed that radiation led to cell death."而"We could detect the 80-kD protein⋯". 最好改为:"The 80-kD protein was detected⋯"。

第 10 节　简明原则

写作时最重要的是表达清楚。

尽管学术英语倾向于使用被动语态,但主动语态的使用通常更短更清晰。此外,两种句式的重点不一样。

比较:Galileo discovered the moons of Jupiter.

The moons of Jupiter were discovered by Galileo.

在第一种情况下,重点是伽利略,在第二种情况下(被动)是卫星。

虽然使用短句使表达清楚,但太多的短句会非常单调。因此好的写作通常长句和短句的结合使用。

遵循用最少的字数来表达观点的原则,如许多短语可以用一个单词代替。比如:

➢ to→ in order to

➢ can→ has the capability of

➢ in fact→ As a matter of fact

➢ currently→ at the present time

➢ adequately→in an adequate manner

➢ because, since →due to the fact that

➢ therefore→in view of the foregoing circumstances

➢ rapidly→ at a rapid rate(The infection is spreading rapidly.)

➢ by →by means of(The tumor was diagnosed by radiography.)

➢ many →a large number of(Many students were tested for the virus.)

➢ although, though →in spite of the fact that,despite the fact that

➢ before →prior to(Patient consent was obtained before the study.)

➢ agree →are in agreement(These results agree with previous findings.)

➢ indicate→ are indicative of(The pathological findings indicate metastasis.)

➢ except→with the exception of(All cell types were stained except fibroblasts.)

➢ possibly →it is possible that(Possibly, there was bias in participant selection.)

➢ postoperatively → after the operation(The patient was in pain postoperatively)

> preoperatively → before the operation（Ultrasound was performed preoperatively.）

同样避免同义反复（Tautology），如用"consensus"，不用"consensus of opinion"；用"fewer"，不用"fewer in number"。

以下表达方法尽量避免：

> It is clear that…

> It is shown that…

> It can be noticed that…

> It has been found that…

> Regarding this fact that…

> It has to be mentioned that…

> It should however be noted that…

> As can be seen from the figure（table）…

> Based on our experiments（understanding）…

第 11 节　连接词和连接短语

连接词（Linking word）或连接短语（Linking phrase）主要由连接副词组成，用于将一个句子或段落的意思连接到下一个句子。如果它们位于句子的开头，也被称为句子连接词（Sentence connector）；如果它们连接段落，也被称作过渡词（Transition word）。连接词的目的是帮助读者沿着作者的思路阅读文章，使阅读更加顺畅。

常用的链接词有：

> 举例：as shown by, e. g. , especially, for example, for instance, in particular, namely, particularly, specifically, such as, that is, to illustrate。

> 重复和递进：again, and, also, besides, equally important, first（second, etc.）, further, furthermore, in addition, in the first place, moreover, next。

注意：first, second, third… 或 firstly, secondly, thirdly 都可以用，但不能混搭。

> 类比：also, in the same manner, in the same way, likewise, similarly。

> 对比：although, and yet, at the same time, but, despite, even though, except, however, in contrast, in spite of, nevertheless, on the contrary, on the other hand, regardless of, still, though, unlike, whereas,

yet，instead of，at least。

> 逻辑关系：accordingly, as a result, because, consequently, for this reason, hence, if, otherwise, since, so, then, therefore, thus, owing to, unless, in the event that, for the purpose, under these circumstances。

> 时间关系：after, afterward, as, as long as, as soon as, at last, before, during, earlier, finally, formerly, immediately, later, meanwhile, next, since, shortly, subsequently, then, thereafter, until, when, while。

> 空间关系：adjacent to, above, below, beyond, close, elsewhere, here, nearby, opposite, to the right, left, north, east, south, west, etc。

> 总结：in conclusion, in summary, on the whole, that is, therefore, to conclude, to sum up。

如果在从句开头使用连接词，它们应该后跟逗号。在子句的中间，连接词的前后都要放逗号。通过变换使用链接词可增加文章的可读性。

此外，也可用链接句子，如："This has four consequences. First, … "或 "This can be illustrated by the following example"。

第 12 节　代　词

代词（例如 it、them、these、which、who 等）用于指代名词（代词的先行词）。如果先行词在前一句中，代词的使用可能有助于增加句子之间的关系。然而，代词应明确其所指代的先行词。例如："The method was applied in an experiment. It consisted of three steps."是模棱两可的，无法判断"It"到底是指"method"还是"experiment"。如果是指"experiment"，应该改为"The method was applied in an experiment that consisted of three steps. "

第 13 节　平行结构

平行结构（parallel structure）包括明显具有相同语法模式的重复句子或重复短语。一系列连续句子中的重复模式有助于读者判断句子之间的联系。平行结构可以应用于单词、短语或从句，通常通过使用"and"或"or"等协调连词连接。例如：

> In spring, summer, or winter.

> A slope failure results in transport of debris downhill by slumping, sliding, rolling, or falling.

> The sinking of deltas causes coasts to recede, water levels to rise, and salt water to intrude further landward.

注意,平行结构应该是相同的语法形式,以便它们是平行的。所以,避免以下做法:

> In spring, summer, or in winter.

> A slope failure results in transport of debris downhill by slumping, sliding, rolling, or by rockfall.

> The sinking of deltas causes coasts to recede, water levels to rise, and landward intrusion of salt water.

第14节　同义词的使用

一篇论文中关键词要保持一致,避免在论文中使用关键词的同义词。另一方面,通过使用同义词来表示等同的意思,避免过度使用关键字以外的单词。要查找合适的同义词,可以使用同义词库(例如:www. thesaurus. com)。

第15节　动词时态和语态

在科学写作中,动词时态的正确使用有一些约定。除了遵循时间(过去、现在、将来)之外,论文中使用的动词时态还可以揭示出谁的想法(你的或他人的)以及描述的事情是普遍的还是特别具体的。

一般现在时(simple present)用于描述现在或定期发生的动作。在科学论文中,这个时态用于描述普遍接受的科学事实或自己的陈述。因此,它通常应用于前言部分对主要观点进行文献综述或陈述。结果部分呈现图表内容的时候也用现在时,例如:"Figure 3 shows that…"。

过去时用于描述过去的研究(如前言中),包括您正在报告的自己的研究(方法和结果)。

现在完成时用于描述从过去开始并持续到现在的未完成动作。在科学论文中,这种时态的使用通常仅限于引言部分(文献综述),以表明该领域的研究仍在继续或仍具有直接相关性。例如:" Recently, there has been a strong debate about the mechanisms of cell apoptosis. "

被动语态强调所做的事情,通常被认为是更客观的(因此,更"科学"),但也被认为是啰嗦的,而且常常令人厌烦。相反,主动语态被认为更加简洁明了;它恰当地描述了研究者积极开展的研究。传统上,科学论文依赖于被动语态的使用,但现在大多数科学风格的论文支持使用主动语态。一般来说如果不知道谁或什么对行为负责,则用被动语态。

第 16 节　拼　写

尽管英式英语和美式英语在许多方面大体相似,但要注意一些拼写差异。美式英语和英式英语的主要区别在牛津词典网站上可以找到。

如果杂志没有特别指明,论文可选择美式英语或英式英语之一,并在整个论文中保持拼写一致。请注意,参考文献应以原始拼写引用。

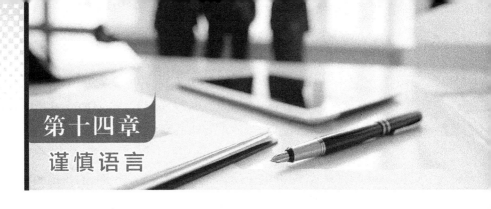

第十四章
谨慎语言

学术写作的一个重要特征就是谨慎语言(Cautious language，Tentative language)的使用。"Cautious language"也称为"Hedging"（回避）或"Vague"（含糊其词）。当引用他人的研究结论时，不同的动词表达的谨慎程度不一样：

➤ Tilic states that the cost of living has increased（表达正面的意思）。

➤ Lee suggests that more research is needed（表达谨慎的意思）。

在医学写作中，对于本研究中不确定的结论，或有例外的结论，一般要采用谨慎用语，避免审稿人误解，尤其是在引言中。如：

➤ Large studies tend to show a relation between duration of smoking and risk of diabetes.

➤ Light smoking seems to have dramatic effects on cardiovascular diseases.

➤ Light smoking might also be associated with a higher than expected risk of cardiovascular diseases.

在讨论中也常用，如：

➤ This study has a few limitations. Firstly, we excluded 25% of the households from analysis because of missing information on either income or BMI. It is unlikely that such missing information is related to price elasticity or purchase behaviour.

"Cautious language"可以采用的方法很多，常用的有：

• 介绍动词：seem，tend，look like，appear to be，think，believe，doubt，indicate，assume，hypothesise 和 suggest。如：Fertility rates tend to fall as societies get richer.

- 情态动词：will, must, would, may, might 和 could。

- 频率副词：often, sometimes, usually。如：Demand for healthcare usually exceeds supply.

- 标示部分的词：to some extent。

- 情态副词：certainly, definitely, clearly, probably, possibly, perhaps, conceivably, roughly, about, reasonably, somehow, somewhat。

- 情态形容词：certain, definite, clear, probable, unlikely, uncertain 和 possible。

- 情态名词：assumption, possibility 和 probability。

- 短语：as a rule, in our opinion, in our view 和 to our knowledge。

- 指出特定条件：in the context of …, … in certain situations …, within some households …

- 从句：

We feel that …

We believe that …

It is our view that …

It has the potential to …

One would expect that …

It could be the case that …

It is important to develop …

It is generally agreed that …

A likely explanation is that …

It may be possible to obtain …

A probable explanation is that …

A possible explanation is that …

- 在形容词前面使用 quite, rather 或者 fairly。如：a fairly accurate summary; a rather inconvenient method; quite a significant discovery。quite 通常表达积极的结果，而 rather 则倾向于表达消极的结果。

有些用法之间可以互换：

appear to be → apparently(*adv*)

assume → assumption(*n*)

estimate → estimation(*n*)

doubt→doubtful(*adj*)

indicate→indication(*n*)

likely→likelihood(*n*)

probably→probable(*adj*)→probability(*n*)

possibly→possible(*adj*)→possibility(*n*)

seem to→seemingly(*adv*)

tend to→tendency(*n*)

医学论文中需要用到谨慎语言的地方有：

(1) 概述需要检验的假设(例如在引言中)。

(2) 讨论一项还不能完全肯定的研究的结果。

(3) 评论其他研究者的研究。

(4) 做出预测(通常用"may"或"might")。

常用的句子：

• 表明自己对某个观点有保留意见时,可以用以下句式：

According to X, …

It is thought that …

It is believed that …

X holds the view that …

It has been reported that …

It is a widely held view that …

If X's findings are accurate, …

According to recent reports, …

According to many in the field …

It has commonly been assumed that …

Recent research has suggested that …

There is some evidence to suggest that …

• 解析某个结果时,可以用以下句式：

A possible explanation for this might be that …

It seems possible that these results are due to …

This rather contradictory result may be due to …

The observed increase in X could be attributed to …

The possible interference of X cannot be ruled out …

There are several possible explanations for this result.

There are two likely causes for the differences between…

This inconsistency may be due to(could be attributed to) …

A possible explanation for these results may be the lack of adequate…

Since this difference has not been found elsewhere it is probably not due

to…

• 提出某个可能有瑕疵的结果时,可以用以下句式:

These data must be interpreted with caution because…

These results therefore need to be interpreted with caution.

These results do not rule out the influence of other factors in…

It is important to bear in mind the possible bias in these responses.

However, with a small sample size, caution must be applied, as the

findings might not be…

• 讨论某个结果的意义时,可以用以下句式:

One possible implication of this is that…

Taken together, these results suggest that…

The evidence from this study suggests that…

The findings of this study(Initial observations) suggest that…

The data reported here appear to support the assumption that…

• 讨论某个建议时,可以用以下句式:

Strategies to enhance X might involve…

These results would seem to suggest that the…

There would therefore seem to be a definite need for…

A reasonable approach to tackle this issue could be to…

Another possible area of future research would be to investigate why…

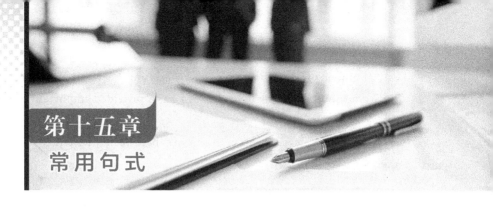

第十五章 常用句式

　　一般认为一篇论文中同一种词汇和相同的句子尽量不要重复使用,尤其是在同一个段落中。因此要掌握不同的句式。

1. 引入主题的常用句式

Regarding X, …

In terms of X, …

In the case of X …

With regard to X, …

With respect to X, …

On the question of X, …

As far as X is concerned, …

A primary concern of X is …

X has(plays) a vital role …

X is frequently prescribed for …

Xs have been extensively used for …

X is an increasingly important area in …

X is a major area of interest within the field of …

X has received considerable attention since …

X has been studied by many researchers using …

X is one of the most widely used immunosuppressants and …

X has long been a question of great interest in the field of …

It is now well established from a variety of studies that X is …

Evidence suggests that X is among the most important factors for …

Recently several investigators examined the effects of X on Y and found …

There is a growing body of literature that recognises the importance of …

A number of studies suggest an association between X and Y…

Studies over the past two decades have provided important information on…

A considerable amount of literature has been published on X. These studies…

2. 突出时间节点的常用句式

Recently, there has been renewed interest in…

In recent years, there has been an increasing interest in…

Recent developments in the field of X have led to a renewed interest in…

The last two decades have seen a growing trend towards…

Over the past decade, there has been a dramatic increase in…

The past decade has seen the rapid development of X in many…

Since it was reported in 2020, X has been attracting much interest.

The past thirty years have seen increasingly rapid advances in the field of…

注意,不用"nowadays",用"presently"或"currently"。不用"(up) until now",用"to date"。

3. 提出问题,或指出某一研究的不足

X is a major problem in…

Of particular concern is…

One of the main obstacles…

One of the greatest challenges…

The main disadvantage of X is that…

There is increasing concern that…

The main limitation of X, however, is…

Previous studies of X have not dealt with…

Previous published studies are limited to…

One major drawback of this approach is that…

It is now well established that X can impair…

Most studies have only a small number of patients.

Half of the studies failed to demonstrate whether…

Most studies in the field of X have only focused on…

Such approaches, however, have failed to address…

Selection bias is another potential concern because…

This approach has various well known limitations.

This method does involve potential measurement error.

Half of the studies evaluated failed to specify whether…

X is one of the most frequently reported side effects with…

However，this method of analysis has a number of limitations.

X's analysis does not take account of…，nor does she examine…

Previously published studies on the effect of X are not consistent.

Exposure to X has been shown to be related to adverse effects in…

All the studies reviewed so far，however，suffer from the fact that…

Another problem with this approach is that it fails to take X into account.

These short-term studies do not necessarily show changes over time.

The existing stidues fail to resolve the contradiction between X and Y.

One of the limitations with this study is that it does not explain why…

Although extensive research has been carried out，no single study exists which…

The generalisability of published clinical studies on this treatment strategy is problematic.

However，these results were based upon data from over 20 years ago and it is unclear if…

However，all the previously mentioned methods suffer from some serious drawbacks(limitations、weaknesses、shortcomings 或 disadvantages).

4. 对他人的研究的评价和意见

X has also questioned why…

However, X points out that…

We challenges the widely held view that…

The idea that… was first challenged by X.

However, we question this hypothesis and…

In a recent article，X questions the extent to which…

Other authors question the efficacy of such a treatment.

X has challenged some of Y's conclusions，arguing that…

A recently published article casts doubt on assumption that…

More recent arguments against X have been summarised by X：

We are critical of the conclusions that Smith draws from his findings.

In her discussion of X，Y further criticises the ways in which some authors …

The X theory has been vigorously challenged in recent years by a number of studies.

Many studies have also argued that not only do previous studies provide an inaccurate measure of X, but the …

5. 指出过去缺乏相关研究

However，X may cause …

However，X is limited by …

It is still not known whether …

There is little published data on …

Currently，there are no data on …

However，a major problem with X is …

No previous study has investigated X.

The use of X has not been investigated.

There has been no large-scale studies of …

However，the study fails to consider that …

Research to date has not yet determined …

What is not yet clear is the impact of X on …

There is still uncertainty，however，whether …

However，X suffers from many disadvantages …

However，X is too expensive to be used for …

However，the performance of X is limited by …

The response of X to Y is not fully understood.

However，X is associated with increased risk of …

Data about the efficacy and safety of X are limited.

The neurobiological basis of X is poorly understood.

However，there is an inconsistency with this argument.

However，they fails to acknowledge the significance of …

However，the influence of X on Y has remained unclear.

A research of the literature revealed few studies which …

In addition，no research has been found that surveyed …

However，research has consistently shown that X lacks …

So far，very little attention has been paid to the role of X …

The mechanisms that underpin X are not fully understood.

However, current methods of X have proven to be unreliable.

However, the author overlooks the fact that X contributes to…

However, the author makes no attempt to differentiate between…

However, the main weakness of the study is the failure to address how…

However, the availability of vaccines remains a major challenge.

A systematic understanding of how X contributes to Y is still lacking.

Much uncertainty still exists about the relationship between…

There have been no controlled studies which compare differences between…

To date, there are few studies that have investigated the association between…

However, the research does not take into account the patients' pre-existing conditions such as…

However, the author did not analyse how(ascertain whether, distinguish between, explain the meaning of, provide information on, address the question of, assess the effectiveness of, consider the long term impact of, determine the underlying causes of)…

6. 提出一个争议性问题

One major issue in X is…

A much debated question is whether…

The issue of X has been a controversial…

To date there has been little agreement on what…

Questions have been raised about the use of X in…

Researchers have long debated the impact of X on…

In the literature, the relative importance of Y is debated.

Debate continues about the best strategies for the management of…

This concept has recently been challenged by studies demonstrating…

More recently, literature has emerged that offers contradictory findings about…

The causes of X have been the subject of intense debate within the scientific community.

The experimental data are rather controversial, and there is no general agreement about…

In the literature, the relative importance of X has been subjected to considerable discussion.

7. 引出本研究的目的

To compare the difference between…

hanges in X and Y were compared using…

The specific objective of this study was to…

Regression analysis was used to predict the…

To distinguish between these two possibilities,…

This case study examined the changing nature of…

The correlation between X and Y was tested using…

The objectives of this research was to determine whether…

The average scores of X and Y were compared in order to…

In order to assess Z, repeated-measures ANOVAs were used.

The aim of this study was to explore the relationship between…

This prospective study was designed to investigate the effects of…

This research examined the emerging role of X in the context of…

The main aim of this study was to investigate the differences between X and Y.

This study attempted(intended, aimed) to show(determine, unravel) that…

There were two primary aims of this study: 1. To investigate… 2. To ascertain…

This study therefore set out to investigate the usefulness of(assess the effect of X)…

The purpose of this investigation was to explore the relationship between X and Y.

也可以写成：

In this study, we　　compared…

proposed a new treatment for…

examined the relationship between…

investigated the factors that determine…

"However","Despite","While","Whilst"和"Although"是最常用的引出问题的词（注意"However"后面要的逗号）。

While(Whilst,Although) some research has been carried out on X, no single study exists which… (no studies have been found which; no controlled studies have been reported; the mechanism has not been established).

如下段，用现在完成时引出一个现状，然后用"however"引出问题。

➤ Prevention of cytomegalovirus (CMV) infection after hematopoietic stem cell and solid organ transplants has improved immensely in recent years. However, despite clinical advancements in CMV prevention, the development of resistant and refractory CMV infections remains a major complication for post-transplant patients.

8. 介绍过去的事件时候，为了突出对目前研究的影响，常常用现在完成时

Several studies have revealed that…

Previous studies of X have not dealt with…

Until recently, there has been little interest in X.

Since 1900, four papers on X have been published.

To date, little evidence has been found associating X with Y.

A considerable amount of literature has been published on X.

Recently, these questions have been addressed by researchers.

There have been several investigations into the causes of sepsis.

The past decade has seen the rapid development of X in many…

Over the past 30 years there has been a significant increase in…

So far, three factors have been identified as being potentially important.

In recent years, researchers have investigated a variety of approaches to…

More recently, literature has emerged that offers contradictory findings about…

The relationship between a high-fats diet and poor health has been widely investigated…

9. 表达因果关系的句式

X is a key factor in…

X is a major influence on…

X has a positive effect on…

X has a significant impact on…

X has contributed to the decline in…

A number of factors are known to affect…

One reason why Xs have declined is that…

In the literature, X has been associated with Y.

X is an important determinant(driving factor) of…

A consequence of vitamin A deficiency is blindness.

X is generally seen as a factor strongly related to Y.

The causal role of X in Y has been demonstrated by…

This suggests a weak link may exist between X and Y.

The use of X may be linked to behaviour problems in…

It is now understood that X plays an important role in…

X is a significant contributory factor to the development of…

X can have profound health consequences for older people.

The human papilloma virus is linked to most cervical cancer.

The most likely causes of X are poor diet and lack of exercise.

This work has revealed several factors that are responsible for…

Loneliness has twice the impact on early death as obesity does.

Recent research has revealed that X has a detrimental effect on…

All these factors can impact on the efficiency and effectiveness of…

Many other medications have an influence on cholesterol levels.

Therefore, Consequently, Because of this, As a result(of this), Owing to, as a consequence of, thus, thereby

X is a/an (common/dominant/predictive/important/significant/underlying/contributing/confounding/complicating) risk factor in(for) …

10. 举例时常用的句式

X is a good illustration of…

For example(for instance), …

This is certainly true in the case of…

Another example of what is meant by X is…

This is exemplified in the work undertaken by…

This distinction is further exemplified in studies using…

The prices of medicines, such as mAb, have declined over…

Pavlov found that if a stimulus, for example the ringing of a bell, preceded the food.

Many diseases can result at least in part from stress, including: arthritis, asthma, and migraine.

Young people begin smoking for a variety of reasons. They may, for example，be influenced by TV.

"particularly"，"especially"（前后加逗号），则是突出举例。

"a case in point"是指单个例子：

A few diseases have been successfully eradicated. A case in point is smallpox.

Some can be transmitted without obvious symptoms，this disease being a case in point.

11. 研究对象选择

Criteria for selecting the subjects were as follows：

Primary inclusion criteria for the X participants were…

Eligibility criteria required individuals to have received…

Forty-seven students were recruited from 15 clinics for this study.

Eligible women who matched the selection criteria were identified by…

Only children aged between 10 and 15 years were included in the study.

The participants were divided into two groups based on their performance on…

12. 统计学词汇

The data were normalised using….

Descriptive data were generated for all variables.

Reliability was calculated using Cronbach's alpha.

All analyses were carried out using SPSS，version 20.

Statistical analysis was performed using SPSS software(version 20).

Significance levels were set at the 1% level using the student t-test.

Data management and analysis were performed using SPSS 16.0(2010).

The mean score for the two trials was subjected to multivariate analysis of variance to…

13. 引出图表结果（用现在时）

As shown in Figure 1…

As can be seen from Table 1…

The results of the correlational analysis are shown(set out/presented/summarized) in Table 1.

Table 1(Figure 1) shows (compares，presents，provides，illustrates) an overview of (the experimental data on X，the results obtained from the preliminary analysis of X)。

14. 突出图表中的结果

What stands out in Table 1 is…

It is apparent from Table 1 that very few…

The most interesting aspect of this graph is…

In Fig. 1 there is a clear trend of decreasing…

The differences between X and Y are highlighted in Table 1.

From the chart, it can be seen that the greatest decrease occurred in Group 1…

As Table I shows, there is a significant difference (p = 0.03) between the two groups.

15. 阳性结果的描述

A two-way ANOVA revealed that…

On average, Xs were shown to have…

The results, as shown in Table 1, indicate that…

A positive correlation was found between X and Y.

There was a significant positive correlation between…

There was a significant difference between the groups…

The difference between the X and Y groups was significant.

16. 阴性结果的描述

X appeared to be unaffected by Y.

No increase in X was detected.

No difference greater than X was observed.

No significant differences were found between…

There was no evidence that X has an influence on…

None of these differences were statistically significant.

No significant reduction in X was found compared with placebo.

No significant difference between the two groups was observed.

Overall, X did not affect males and females differently in these measures.

No significant correlation was found between X scores and the Y scores (p =)

A clear benefit of X in the prevention of Y could not be identified in this analysis.

T-tests found no significant differences in mean scores on the X and Y subscales.

17. 突出有意思或意外的结果

Interestingly，X was observed to…

This result was somewhat counterintuitive.

The more surprising correlation is with the…

Surprisingly，only a minority of respondents…

18. 趋势的描述

The graph(Figure 2) shows(reveals) that there has been a(slight/steep/sharp/steady/gradual/marked) fall (rise/drop/decline/increase/decrease) in the number of infections in China since 2000.

What is striking(What stands out/What is interesting/What can be clearly seen) in Table 1(Figure 1) is the growth of(the high rate of/the variability of/the dominance of/the rapid decrease in/the steady decline of/the dramatic decline in/the continual growth of/the difference between)…

19. 最大、最小点的描述

The peak age for committing suicide is 80.

Production of cytokine X peaked after 3 days.

The number of Xs reached a peak(a low point) during(in)…

20. 数量的描述

• 分数

Nearly half of the patients(48%) died.

Half of those surveyed did not comment on…

The number of patients fell by nearly two-fifths.

Over(Approximately) half of those enrolled were male.

Less than a third of those who responded(32%) indicated that…

Of the 148 patients who completed the treatment，just over half reported side effects.

Well over (More than/Just over/Around/Almost/As many as/Approximately/Just under/Less than/Fewer than/Well under) half(a third/

a quarter/ XX%) of those treated (of the patients/of those who were treated) recovered…

- 比例

Group 1 has the highest proportion of male patients.

The response rate was 60% at six months and 56% at 12 months.

The annual birth rate dropped from 44. 4 to 38. 6 per 1000 per annum.

Scotland had the lowest proportion of lone parents at only 14 per cent.

The proportion of live births outside marriage reached one in ten in 1945.

The proportion of the population attending emergency departments was 65%.

Since 1981, England has experienced an 89% increase in infection of HIV.

With each year of advancing age, the probability of having dementia increased by 9. 6%.

The mean income of the bottom 20 percent of families declined from $10,000 in 1970 to $8,000 in 1976.

They found that of 2,500 abortions, 58% were in young women aged 15 – 24, of whom 62% were black.

- 平均数

The mean age of patients with coronary atherosclerosis was 48. 3 ± 6. 3 years.

Mean estimated age at death was 80. 1 ± 12. 0 years(ranging from 70. 3 to 90. 3 years).

They had smoked for an average of 15 years(range 6 to 20 years).

- 范围和大约数

The participants were aged 19 to 25.

Estimates of death range from 200,000 to 700,000 and up to a million or more.

Rates of decline ranged from 2. 71 – 0. 08 cms per day with a mean of 0. 97 cm per day.

The evidence shows that survival time from cancer diagnosis lies in the range of twenty to thirty years.

虽然数字代表精准,但太多数字会让文章读起来枯燥。 如果数字不是很重要,这时候可以用代表数字趋势的词汇(表 15.1)。

表 15.1　数字趋势词汇

词	意思
few	比想象的少
a few	大约 3～6
several	大约 3～4
various	大约 4～6
dozens	大约 30～60
scores	60～100
a tiny/small minority	5%～20%
a minority	21%～39%
a substantial/significant minority	40%～49%
a small majority	51%～55%
a majority	56%～79%
a large majority	80%

其他表达方法还有:

one in three patients was treated

a quarter/fifth of patients were male

a small/large proportion of the patients

the highest(lowest) rate of death was in

twice as many female as male have lupus

the majority/ minority of births are in hospital

the rate of infection halved(doubled) after 2001

there was a fivefold increase in the number of patients

21. 比较的修饰词

slightly, considerably, significantly and substantially, substantially larger than, slightly smaller than, significantly older than。

half as large as, twice as large as, ten times as fast as。

• 介绍差异:

By contrast, In contrast, On the other hand, In contrast to, Compared with, differ from, contrast with, different from

22. 讨论中的总结

These results suggest that…

Overall, these results indicate that…

In summary, these results show that…

Together, the study indicates that…

Considering all of this evidence, it seems that…

The evidence study suggests that…

Taken together, the study supports the notion that…

The study supports the hypothesis that…

Together the study(these results) provides important insights into…

Taken together, these results suggest that there is an association between…

The study clearly indicates that there is a relationship between…

Collectively, the study outlines a critical role for…

总结的句子一般用复数,"the"＋单数是比较正式的方法。对于可能有例外的情况的总结,可以加标示倾向性的词汇。如:

➢ Computers have transformed the way we live.

➢ The computer has transformed the way we live.

➢ Young children tend to learn second languages easily.

总结一般使用谨慎语言。使用"show"、"demonstrate"和"suggest",不要用"prove"。

除非特别重要的发现,不要用"for the first time"或"wholly explains"。

在讨论一些常识性的东西的时候,用谨慎语言,如:

➢ It is generally accepted that…

➢ It is widely agreed that…

➢ It is probable that…

➢ The evidence suggests that…

23. 讨论中突出研究的重要性词汇

This is the first RCT study to…

This study provides new insights into…

This work generates fresh insight into…

The importance of this study is that it explores…

The study offers some important insights into…

Understanding the link between X and Y will help…

The present research explores, for the first time, the effects of…

The experimental work presented here provides one of the first investigations into how…

Therefore, this study makes a major contribution to research on diabetes by demonstrating…

24. 引入关于作者本人的新方法的讨论

In contrast to earlier findings, …

A major advantage of X is that…

The benefit of this approach is that…

X method has a number of advantages over…

X is different from Y in a number of respects.

This method is particularly useful in studying…

X differs from Y in a number of important ways.

The advantages of Xs are that they are simple to deliver.

There are a number of important differences between X and Y.

We found dramatic differences in the rate of X between Y and Z.

One advantage of the X analysis is that it avoids the problem of…

These results are similar to those reported by X et al.

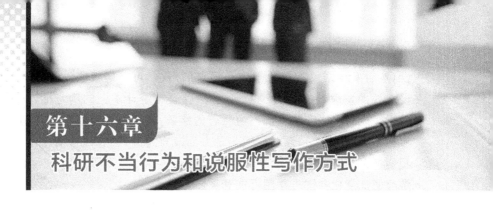

第十六章
科研不当行为和说服性写作方式

在医学领域，研究人员在分析数据和撰写论文时可能会在知情或不知情的情况下违反科学原则。这章我们将介绍一些介于灰色地带的科研不当行为（Questionable research practice，QRP）和需要尽量避免的说服性写作方式（Persuasive communication device）。

第1节　科研不当行为

有些研究人员可能不一定意识到有些行为是科学不端行为，尤其是缺乏经验的年轻人，因此了解这些 QRP 的知识很有必要[1]。现阶段由于很多机构和杂志要求在临床研究开始之前强制性完成在线注册，下述的临床研究 QRP 很少发生了。

HARKING

HARKing 的意思是"在结果已知后进行假设（Hypothesizing After the Results are Known）"。HARKing 是一种 QRP。有些研究人员分析数据后发现一些非预期的、具有统计学意义的结果，然后根据该结果提出新的假设。这个本身没有错误，毕竟科学中的许多重要发现都是在研究结束和检查数据之后偶然发现的。然后如果论文撰写成此项研究是为了检验该假设进行设计、开展和分析的，那就不对了。正确的做法是当在检查结果后做出假设时，应承认分析是探索性的，属于事后假设（Post hoc hypothesis），这个发现可能是偶然发现，需要在未来的研究中得到证实。

HARKing 会误导读者。如果我们在开始研究之前建立假设，然后发现结果在统计学上是显著的，我们可以确信假设是对的。然而预设之外的发现可能是偶然发现，无法保证在统计学上的确定性。

假设我们研究某个抗高血压药的疗效，发现治疗有反应和没有反应的患者在年龄、性别等一系列基线变量方面没有差异，但在反应者中素食者更多。我们可以在讨论中就素食可能通过某些机制产生降压作用，如：果蔬中的黄烷醇的抗氧化和抗炎作用可能和降压有关。

如果把论文撰写成研究素食对血压的影响，并得出结论素食可以降血压，虽然所有的数据都是真的，作者并没有造假，但偶然性甚至是假阳性的结论将被当成了一个科学结论进行传播，并且在主流科学文献中持续存在。这就是一种 QRP

临床试验论文中作者必须确保报告的研究设计和结果与研究人员公布的设计方案保持一致。编辑会仔细审查这些文件，以确保一致性，并确保作者对任何差异提供解释和理由。这也是预防"HARKing"的有效方式。

注意："HARK"可以作为不及物动词。

» CHERRY-PICKING

摘樱桃的人不会选择看起来不好吃的水果，因此"摘樱桃"式的报道指研究人员只选择并报告支持他们假设的内容。例如，研究人员可能会发现在抗抑郁药试验中研究药物在部分抑郁评分表上优于安慰剂。研究人员为此只报告阳性结果的量表，不报告疗效不显著的量表结果。摘樱桃式的报道可以说是欺骗了读者。

除了在原创性研究外，在荟萃分析中作者也可能通过挑选已发表的论文结果来支持或否定他们期望的假设。

» P-HACKING

"P-hacking"指研究人员以不同的方式分析数据，直到获得具有统计学意义的结果。"P-hacking"的目的不是为了检验一个假设，而是为了获得一个重要的结果。为此研究人员用不同的统计方法来检验一个假设；或者改变协变量的种类；或者用不同的截止值进行分析。显然这违背了科学研究的目的，因为研究人员已经提前决定了研究结果，因此属于 QRP。

FISHING EXPEDITIONS，DATA MINING，AND DATA DREDGING

"钓鱼探险(Fishing expedition)"一词指研究人员无目的地检测不同变量组合之间的关联,他们的目的不是为了检验先验假设(Priori hypotheses),而是希望在数据中找到具有统计意义的东西并撰写论文。例如,研究人员可以用每一个可用的结果变量来测试每一个可能预测高血压发生的因素。很明显,由于涉及大量的统计测试,假阳性的风险很高。研究者往往将钓鱼探险和"HARKing"配合使用。

数据挖掘(Data dredging or data mining)属于"Fishing expedition",指研究者对数据库中可用数据的变量之间进行广泛的分析。"P-hacking"和数据挖掘之间的区别在于,"P-hacking"通常指从与一个或多个感兴趣的假设相关的数据中寻找统计显著性,而数据挖掘是在不一定考虑特定假设的情况下,在数据集中广泛搜索统计显著的关系,假阳性结果的概率非常高。

虽然"Data dredging"和"Data mining"的意思相同,在当今的大数据时代,医学研究中数据挖掘是符合伦理的。在这种特定的背景下"Data mining"一词并不是贬义词。"Data dredging"用于描述有 QRP 嫌疑的数据挖掘。

剽窃

剽窃是将他人的文字、思想(设计、理念等)或图像呈现为自己的行为;它没有尊重作者应得的荣誉。无论是有意还是无意,剽窃都违反了学术道德标准。

剽窃者故意避开原创作者的贡献,不尊重原创作者的工作;甚至欺骗读者。

避免被认为剽窃的直接方法是通过引文注明资料的来源。

如果想使用他人的表格、图表和图像,必须获得对方的版权持有人的许可。来自互联网的免费图像或通过知识共享获得的图像也需要注明版权归属。

一般出版商会使用剽窃检查软件(例如,iThenticate、Turnitin)来识别是否有论文复制、指定长度的段落匹配度或是否有"Patchwriting"。

自我剽窃(Self-plagiarism)是指将自己以前发表的作品作为原创作品进行展示;像剽窃一样,自我剽窃也是不道德的。如果论文一稿多投而且发表(Duplicate publication),可能会导致侵犯版权。

通过总结和释义避免剽窃,证明你对原文完全理解。释义(Paraphrasing)指重新编写文本,使语言在内容不变的情况下完全不同。有效的释义通常是结构与原版不同,主要词汇不同,可保留一些常用的原始短语。释义技巧包括使用同义词(argues>claims;eighteenth century>1 700 s。不过有些词没有真正的同义词,不能勉强);改变词类(explanation>explain)和更改词序。

总结(Summarising)意味着减少文本长度,但保留要点。

第2节　说服性写作方式

毫无疑问作者需要依靠一系列的写作手段和技巧来吸引读者的兴趣,并说服他们相信作者的观点或观点有过人之处。作者可以使用各种有说服力的沟通手段来实现这些目标。然而在写一篇科学文章时作者必须小心使用这些说服性的写作方式(Persuasive communication device)[2]。作者必须明确自己的研究的局限性,不要过度描述结果(Oversell)。此外也不易用夸大重要性和/或掩盖弱点的方法。当研究人员对科学知识的现状做出不准确的陈述时,他们有可能在研究的新颖性或强度方面误导读者。常见的说服性写作方式有:

- 故意忽略前人的工作或类似结果的文章,担心降低当前研究的新颖性。
- 片面引用支持性研究,忽略不支持作者观点的研究或与自己的研究结果不一致的文章。
- 文章中的观点或证据没有相关引文支持。
- 临床研究在没有进一步证据支持的情况下,武断地将研究结果推广到所研究的人群之外。
- 过度使用夸大结论的形容词,如"striking","important","remarkable","outstanding","excellent"和"unprecedented"。
- 断章取义地引用其他作品以表明观点,包括夸大和歪曲他人研究的结论,以支持自己的结果。
- 故意提供大量、杂乱的研究数据作为补充材料,给审稿人增加审稿难度。
- 相对多描写轻微的局限性,对研究的严重局限性轻描淡写,甚至隐瞒。
- 对具有不同或相互竞争观点的研究者,希望对方提供更高标准的证据。
- 对有已知缺陷的方法,试图通过强调它已经在以前的许多研究中使用过而证明采用该方法的合理性。

- 将不符合作者标准的知名科学家列入作者，以增加稿件被接受的机会。

- 使用夸大的标题来吸引读者。

- 采用晦涩的词汇。例如，"influence"一词可以用来暗示因果关系，而不必明确声称因果关系已经得到证明，从而在另一位研究人员对这一发现提出疑问时为作者提供了回旋余地。

这里列出的问题并不一定源于作者故意误导读者的意图。例如对有些相关工作没有描写可能是因为受到参考文献数量的限制。此外作者可能参考了其他人的论文的内容，没有进行独立的文献调研。无论如何我们要认真对待论文写作，避免对研究结果的误解和对科学带来的有害影响。

参考文献

[1] Andrade C. HARKing, cherry-picking, P-hacking, fishing expeditions, and data dredging and mining as questionable research practices[J]. J Clin Psychiatry,2021,82(1):20f13804.

[2] O Corneille, Jo Havemann, E L HendersonHans, et al. IJzermanIan HusseyJean-Jacques Orban de XivryLee JussimNicholas P HolmesArtur PilacinskiBrice BeffaraHarriet CarrollNicholas Otieno OutaPeter LushLeon D Lotter(2023) Point of View:Beware 'persuasive communication devices' when writing and reading scientific articles[EB/OL]. https://apastyle. apa. org/style-grammar-guidelines/grammar/singular-they.

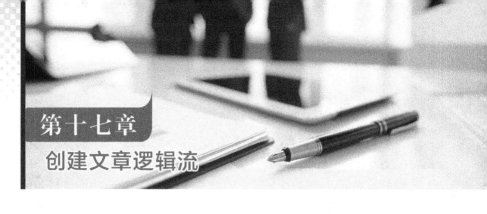

第十七章
创建文章逻辑流

　　在英文中逻辑意味着推理、讲道理,体现的是前后和因果关系(Both logic and logistics ultimately derive from the Greek logos, meaning "reason".[1])。"flow"的定义是"a smooth uninterrupted movement or progress"[2],因此其内涵是稳定和连续。而作为重要的写作技巧,"逻辑流"(logical flow)指在写作时使读者从一句话到下一句话,从一段话到另一段话能够流畅地阅读。就像读者跟随你的思想在小溪上一边缓缓漂流,一边欣赏两岸的风光。句子的流畅性也是如此。你的思路不能大起大落,突然停止并跳跃到另外一个主题上。读者想要一个愉快的、不用费力猜测你的思路的旅程,因此写作需要遵循逻辑流的原则。保持思路清晰,以简洁的方式写作,将术语、语言、事实和观点编织成一个高度连贯的信息。文章内容杂乱无章会严重影响审稿人对内容的注意力,甚至被拒稿。

　　创建文章逻辑流主要有三种方式:

　　(1)内容的逻辑布局,坚持"一个段落一个观点"的原则(one idea-one paragraph principle)。

　　(2)恰当地使用过渡将段落融合在一起。当内容变化的时候采用过渡短语把两行或两段连接起来。

　　(3)保持文体、语气、时态和标点的一致性,如"The important thing for us is to be able to channel one's anxiety into positive action"应该改为"The important thing for us is to be able to channel <u>our</u> anxiety into positive action"。

　　在前面的章节中,我们陆陆续续介绍了一些创建文章逻辑流的方法,如段落的结构、过渡词、单词代替词组、前言的漏斗结构等等。下面我们将继续介绍一些方法。

➤➤ 写出清晰的句子

句子的清晰性决定了文章的可读性和可理解性。要写出清晰的句子,首先要专注于一个主题,不要在一个句子中试图表达多个意思。在不牺牲清晰性的前提下,尽量减少句子中间的片段(例如:which, that, although, where, when)。少用修饰语(例如: very, basically, generally),避免以"that", "who"和"which"开头的不必要的从句(如"This is a procedure that is recommended by the FDA"改为"This procedure is recommended by the FDA")。采用不同类型、长度和开头的句子。通过并列的句子把具有相同意思的句子组合起来。通过使用代词,重复关键词,插入过渡词或短语(例如, therefore, however, consequently)将句子中的观点联系起来。

在医学论文中,采用括号注解的方法是使句子简洁的常用方法,如:

"The histological types were distributed and classified as adenocarcinoma in 51 cases, squamous cell carcinoma in 24 cases, and carcinoid in 10 cases."改为 "The histological types were adenocarcinoma ($n=51$), squamous cell carcinoma ($n=24$), and carcinoid ($n=10$)."

"The FIQ score of the tai chi group was decreased by 27.8 points the FIQ score of the control group was decreased by 9.4 points. The tai chi group had a significantly greater decrease in the total FIQ score than did the control group"改为"The tai chi group had a significantly greater decrease in the total FIQ score than did the control group (-27.8 points $vs.$ -9.4 points)".

➤➤ 引言

引言描述该研究如何为解决一个重要问题。引言部分一般用三个段落创建逻辑流。第一段描述目标问题的范围、性质或严重性。第二段清楚地说明为什么更好地理解这个问题是有用的,包括当前的知识和以前研究的局限性。第三段陈述目的并简要解释该研究为科学知识库增加了什么。

➤➤ 方法

准确描述与研究目标或目的相关的数据是如何收集、组织和分析的。首先描述研究设计,其次是研究地点、研究对象、数据收集方法,最后是数据分析。不要在方法部分写部分结果。

结果

首先设计图以揭示数据趋势或关系,然后起草表格以显示特定的数据。在描述主要结果时,使用这些图和表格作为支持证据。接下来用尽量少的文字和句子总结每个图和表格。记得要连接好各个部分。

讨论

讨论是一篇科学文章的基石,务必写得准确、简洁和没有歧义。为了实现逻辑流畅可以分为 4~6 个段落。第一段简要重申研究的目的或目标是什么、强调关键的结果,重点是这些结果是如何支持了研究目标。第二段、第三段和第四段将每个关键结果与相关文献联系起来。在解释关键结果时,要强调它们的创新性、价值和相关性。通过评估这些新数据提示现在可以实现什么,或者可以填补哪些以前的知识空白。在讨论关键结果时遵循方法和结果相同的顺序。第五段列出研究的优点。第六段说明方法、结果的局限性。最后陈述研究的结论和含义。就本研究需要改进的地方提出建议。描述需求并提出未来研究的展望。

总之,掌握创建逻辑流的方法非常重要,但需要时间。作为为读者创造轻松阅读的关键因素,时间和汗水是值得的。

参考文献

[1] Merriam-webster. Flow[EB/OL]. https://www.merriam-webster.com/dictionary/flow.

[2] Merriam-webster. Logic [EB/OL]. https://www.merriam-webster.com/dictionary/logic.

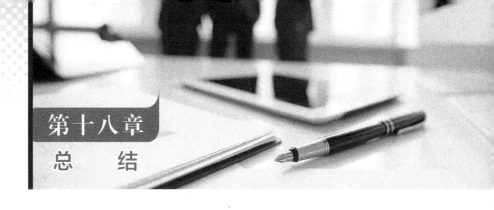

第十八章 总结

年轻的研究人员常常满怀热情地开展研究,完成数据收集和分析,最终得出答案。但当他们第一次尝试撰写论文时,他们的热情却逐渐减弱。在世界范围会议上发表的摘要数量远远超过最终发表在医学文献中的论文数量。未能将好作品出版的部分原因是缺乏经验的研究者在写作的时候遇到很多困惑。然而,撰写研究论文在很大程度上是公式化的,一旦对论文结构有了深入的理解,写作的流程将更加简单。

一、论文撰写

论文撰写的步骤大概如下:

1. 决定写论文

没有什么比坚持和决心更重要。记住写论文对你的职业至关重要,对你的晋升至关重要。

2. 与指导老师交流

在开始写作之前,确保写作方向是正确的。和指导老师在假设、数据分析和解释上充分讨论,达成一致意见。指导老师能够对研究做出合理的评估,并推荐合适的目标期刊。早期确定目标期刊可以让你在写作时按照该期刊的指南来编排论文的格式。

3. 创建时间表

(1)读文献,做笔记,建立模板文件,设定完成日期:文献检索应至少持续 2 个月。按相关性排序收集文章。找出两三篇很相关的文章,仔细阅读这些文章,借鉴他们的写作思路。使用这些文章作为自己的论文模板对理顺自己的思路非常有帮助。关注这些文章中包含的参数和变量作为自己的研究的参考。特别感兴趣的段落或词句可参考使用,但不能抄袭。

(2)为论文设计大纲和标题:在大纲中,不要太详细。可以不写完整句子,只写短语。

(3)起草初稿:按照漏斗原则写引言,确保第一段和最后一段对读者有吸引力。注意方法和结果的第一句。讨论的第一段与最后一段也非常重要。准备表格和图表。

初稿最难,作者往往会觉得很难达到自己预定的标准。目标不要太高,尽快写完。最终结果很可能是一份粗糙、杂乱无章、令人失望的草稿,但这是一个完全令人满意的开始。

按照以下纲领再次核对前言和讨论是否写得充分:

表 18.1　核对表格

前言	1. 概述研究领域
	2. 指出先前研究中的问题
	2a 本研究以解决具体问题为目的?
	2b 本研究以增加现有知识为目的?
	3. 提出新的研究目的
讨论	4. 突出研究结果
	4a 是否明确主要发现
	4b 讨论具体结果,是否通过和参考文献的先前研究,展现本研究的新发现、新知识
	4c 有没有解释意外或不满意的结果
	5a 是否有强调本研究的优势
	5b 有没有描写研究的局限性
	6. 总结

我们前面说过,前言的展开好像是漏斗,讨论的展开像倒漏斗,两者合并则像沙漏,互相对应。

(4)第 1 次修订:完成第一稿后,你应该把它放一天,然后重新阅读,问自己以下问题:① 是否完全回答了研究的问题? ② 论文的不同部分字数是否平衡? ③ 讨论是否清晰且合乎逻辑? ④ 有没有遗忘其他要点?

修改工作是一项系统修剪任务。在编辑过程中,你必须愿意为了论文连贯性而删除你喜欢的华丽辞藻。这是一项细致的工作,最好连贯完成。不断重新排序、画箭头、划掉一些句子,增加一些句子。

(5)第 2 次修订。

(6)第 3 次修订,然后让其他作者评估。

(7)根据他人的建议修改。有时候你的合著者会提供你没有想到的讨论内容,或提出建议,从而彻底重组你的论点。

（8）准备摘要。

（9）检查所有数字和单位，并与指导老师一起审查。

（10）如果研究早期确定了作者排序，再次确定作者排序。通常，主要作者应该是第一作者，指导老师应该是最后一位。其他合著者按其贡献程度依次排列在第一作者之后。

二、投稿

当你认为你的论文足够好的时候就投稿。不要追求完美，否则你永远不会把论文寄出去。

临床研究获得审稿人青睐的常见原因是：

- 针对当前需要解决的临床问题；
- 研究设计合理，方法得当；
- 书写良好，逻辑性强，易于理解。

但仅有这三点还不够。要提高被接受的机会还要避免以下错误：

1. 缺乏对现有研究的了解

在前言中你必须证明你非常了解所在领域的问题，并通过相关文献说明这些问题的存在，甚至包括一周前发表的研究。因此需要进行彻底的文献回顾，不遗余力。务必找到每一项类似的研究，尤其是在有影响力的杂志上发表的，并解释为什么你的研究更好或不同，或者你的研究增加了相关的知识。

2. 解释不清楚你为什么做这项研究

需要用非常简单的语言解释一下你为什么进行研究。许多研究者往往不太清楚为什么要这么做，只知道导师让我这么做！所以如果你不确定，一定问清楚，直到你真的明白，并能用一段话解释清楚。

虽然非英语母语的研究者很难写出完美的英语，但准确、有效的语言使用和严密的逻辑结构是基本技能。因此如果对文章结构的合理性没有把握，不妨先写中文，中文底稿完美后再翻译成英文。

3. 不明确期刊的目的和范围

仔细阅读杂志的"Aim and Scope"。最好是目标杂志有发表您的相关研究。如果你不确定，给编辑发送含有标题和摘要的电子邮件，问问你的研究是否属于他们的杂志范围。

4. 没有充分利用"Cover Letter"

"Cover Letter"是你推销研究成果的机会，告诉主编，为什么对目标读者很重要（目标读者要明确指出，如护士、专科医生或全科医生）。它填补了哪些知识空白？它将如何改变临床实践？它会被高引用吗？

5．未能严格遵守杂志要求

必须遵守规则。参考文献的风格不正确，正文字数太多，摘要格式错误，参考文献太多可能都是被即时拒绝的因素。

6．结构欠佳

文章逻辑性强，易于理解很重要。审稿人和编辑都是忙碌的人，他们不可能花太多时间试图理解你的意思。你的写作要清晰简洁，这一点非常重要。

7．未能解决与你的研究相矛盾的问题

不要忽略其他研究人员的相同或类似工作但结果不同的论文。审稿软件会提供相关文献的链接，审稿人也会进行文献检索，以检查你的作品是否原创。确保你在讨论中提到所有相关文献，即使它们与你的工作相冲突。

The secret of getting ahead is getting started.

—Mark Twain

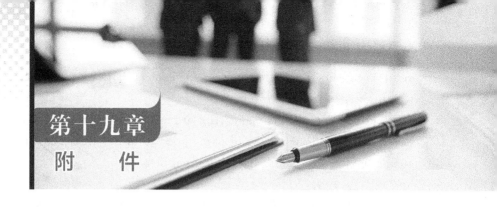

第十九章
附件

Cover Letter 模板

［Date］
Journal Editor-in-Chief ［including title］
Journal Name
Mailing Address(Suite ＃)
City，State，Zip Code
Dear Dr. / Mr. / Ms. Abc：

第一段，介绍文章的题目、类别：On behalf of my colleagues, I would like to submit to "杂志名字"this manuscript of original clinical research(review article，case report，etc.) entitled "稿件题目".

第二段，指出编辑和审稿人可能感兴趣的关键点。可以从论文的引言中摘抄，描述目的、内容、发现和价值，包括一句总结结果的句子，例如：This disease/condition has no current standard of care and this manuscript reports the first randomized clinical findings for this disease.

临床研究说明是否符合临床试验研究的所有国家和国际监管指南(赫尔辛基、EMEA、FDA 等的声明)。

第三段，注明：

The manuscript has been read and approved by all authors. All persons listed as authors have contributed to preparing the manuscript and/or that International Committee of Medical Journal Editors(ICMJE) criteria for authorship have been met， and that no person or persons other than the authors listed have contributed significantly to its preparation.

The contents of this manuscript are my/our original work and have not been published, in whole or in part, prior to or simultaneous with my/our submission of the manuscript to [journal name].

第四段,注明:

详细说明所报告工作的任何资金,以及在写稿过程中的财务或其他支持(包括编辑/写作协助)。例如:The study was funded by XXX Pharmaceuticals. Medical writing services from XXX were funded by XXX Pharmaceuticals.

在适当的情况下应包含与提交的工作相关的商业或公司利益关系产生的任何潜在利益冲突(财务或其他方面)的摘要。例如:This study was funded by a grant from[company]. Authors AA, BB, and CC are or were employees of [company] when this study was conducted and own stock in [company]. Authors DD, EE, and FF received research funding from [company]. Author GG has no conflict of interest to report. We attest that we have herein disclosed any and all financial or other relationships that could be construed as a conflict of interest and that all sources of financial support for this study have been disclosed and are indicated in the acknowledgments.

第五段,描述提交的内容,通常按照期刊说明进行(例如:per journal's instructions, the manuscript and figures, study protocol, author checklist, journal submission form, are included)。

注明是否有任何先前出版的图表,在这种情况下,应包括出版商书面许可的文件。

期刊可能会接受被推荐和被否定的审稿人的建议,这些建议可以在此处列出,也可以在单独的表格中列出。提供所有建议的审稿人的姓名、机构、地址、联系电话和电子邮件。

第六段,包括衷心感谢编辑花时间审阅投稿。

最后是致敬语和签名。目前因为一般都是以电子文档的方式提交,因此传统的手写签名也可以用打印的方式。

以下是2个范本,供参考:

示例1：

August 26, 2011
        Dr. Howard Bauchner, M. D.
        Editor-in-Chief, JAMA

Dear Dr. Bauchner：

Enclosed please find a manuscript entitled "Induction therapy with autologous mesenchymal stem cells in living-related kidney transplantation: a prospective open-label randomized study" for your consideration for publication in JAMA.

In the last couple of years, the therapeutic potential of mesenchymal stem cells in clinical organ transplantation has been investigated yielding promising results in a number of preclinical and pilot clinical studies.

In the enclosed manuscript, we summarize the preliminary result of a prospective, open controlled, randomized clinical study aimed at evaluating the safety and efficacy of autologous mesenchymal stem cells(aMSC) as an immune induction treatment alternative to anti-ILR antibody in a population of patients with end-stage renal disease receiving living-related donor kidney transplantation (LRDKT). The study protocol (ClinicalTrials. gov No. NCT00658073) was approved by the institutional review board (IRB) of Fuzhou General Hospital, People's Republic of China; eligible patients were included in this study in accordance with the Declaration of Helsinki and the selection of candidates for kidney donation was based on the 2004 Amsterdam guidelines.

Patients received aMSC plus standard-dose calcineurin inhibitors(CNI), aMSC plus 80% of standard-dose of CNI, or anti-IL2R (Basiliximab) plus standard-dose CNI. We report on a minimum follow-up of one year(range: 13～30 months). Collectively, our data indicates that aMSC represent a safe induction therapy, being associated with fewer incidents and less severe acute rejection(AR) lesions during the first 6 months post-transplantation, as well as faster recovery of renal function. Based on these results, it is conceivable that the management of transplanted patients may be improved by the means of aMSC therapy. We believe that our finding is important and may help to improve outcome of LRDKT. To the best of our knowledge, this is the first report on a large-scale use of aMSC as an induction strategy for transplant recipients in the clinical setting. We feel that the novelty of the approach and the encouraging results are of interest for the readers of JAMA.

All authors have read and agree with the contents of the submission. As corresponding authors for this report, we both had full access to all the data in the study and take responsibility for the integrity of the data and the accuracy of the data analysis. Additionally, none of the authors has financial or other conflicts of interest that might be construed as influencing the results or interpretation of the study. None of the data in this manuscript has been published or presented previously, nor is under consideration elsewhere at the present time.

We hope that you will find our manuscript of sufficient scientific merit for publication in JAMA.

Yours Sincerely,

XXX, M. D.

Professor of Surgery

Distinguished Professor of Medicine

Director, Diabetes Research Institute & Cell Transplant Center,

University of Miami

1450 NW 10th Avenue, Miami, FL 33136

Tel: XXXX, Fax: XXX,

Email: XXXXX@miami. edu

示例2:

Dear Editor:

Please find enclosed a manuscript entitled "XXXX" by XXX et al. for your consideration for publication in Int J Clin Oncol.

Nasopharyngeal carcinoma has the highest incidence in the southeastern part of China, Taiwan, and Hong Kong. It is usually undifferentiated, nonkeratinizing, and sensitive to radiotherapy. When there is local relapse, re-irradiation treatment is inevitably associated with serious complication and decreased quality of life. Previous studies have shown surgical resection offers an alternate treatment option with acceptable morbidity. The limitation of these studies is the small number of patients involved. In this prospective study we evaluated the results of salvage surgery for 71 patients with primary recurrence of nasopharyngeal carcinoma after radiotherapy. Follow-up ranged from 12 to 127 months. The actuarial 1, 2, 3, and 5-year survival were 88.1%, 62.1%, 48.9% and 42.1% respectively. The 1, 2, 3, and 5-year local control rates were 74.6%, 61.9%, 56.3% and 53.5% respectively. There was no surgical mortality. These data further support that demonstrate that advances in skull base surgery make possible the effective control of primary recurrence of nasopharyngeal carcinoma, with acceptable mortality and morbidity. In addition, we show the prognostic factors with a negative effect on survival of recurrent NPC include advanced stage at treatment lymph node metastasis, invasion of skull base and parapharyngeal space and positive margin.

This is a study of the surgical salvage of NPC in a large Asian cohort. It contains our extensive experience and a wealth of information about integrative therapies for NPC.

We state here none of our authors has financial or other conflicts of interest that might be construed as influencing the results or interpretation of our study.

We state here none of the material has been published or is under consideration elsewhere, including the Internet.

We state here all authors have read and agree with the contents of the submission and have contributed substantially to the work.

We sincerely hope that you find this manuscript of sufficient scientific merit for publication in Int J Clin Oncol.

Best Regards.
Sincerely yours,
XXXX

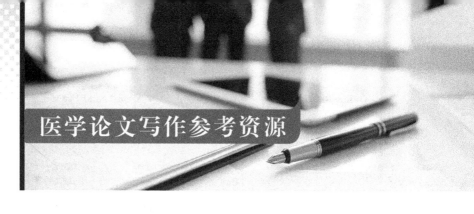

医学论文写作参考资源

Online Resource	Website and Use
JANE	https：//jane. biosemantics. org/ To identify journals and authors with similar articles
Journal Suggester (Taylor and Francis)	https：//authorservices. taylorandfrancis. com/publishing-your-research/choosing-a-journal/ To identify candidate journals
Journal Finder (Elsevier)	https：//journalfinder. elsevier. com/ To identify candidate journals
Journal Suggester (Springer Nature)	journalsuggester. springer. com To identify candidate journals
Journal Finder (Wiley)	https：//journalsuggester. springer. com/ To identify candidate journals
Scimago Journal Rank	https：//www. scimagojr. com/ To identify ranking of journals
NLM Catalog	https：//ncbi. nlm. nih. gov/nlmcatalog To identify indexing of journals
Journal Citation Reports *	https：//jcr. clarivate. com To identify IF of journals
Directory of Open Access Journals	https：//doaj. org/ To identify OA journals
ORCID	https：//orcid. org/ IDs for researchers
Publons	https：//publons. com Information about peer reviewers
Open Science Framework	https：//osf. io/ Data repository

Online Resource	Website and Use
GitHub	https://github.com/ Code repository
figshare	https://figshare.com/ Data repository
Google Scholar	https://scholar.google.com/ Search of citations
Mendeley	https://www.mendeley.com/ Management of references
Zotero	https://www.zotero.org/ Management of references
EndNote *	https://endnote.com/ Management of references
bioRxiv	http://biorxiv.org/ Preprints repository
medRxiv	https://www.medrxiv.org/ Preprints repository
ICMJE recommendations	https://icmje.org/recommendations/browse/ International criteria for writing manuscripts
MeSH on Demand	meshb.nlm.nih.gov/MeSHonDemand Selection of MeSH
Equator Network	https://www.equator-network.org/ Guidelines for reporting
PubPeer	https://pubpeer.com/ To comment on published articles
Retraction Watch	https://retractionwatch.com/ It provides information about retracted articles
Beall's list	https://beallslist.net/ Potential predatory scholarly open-access publishers
COPE	https://publicationethics.org/ Promoting integrity in research and its publication

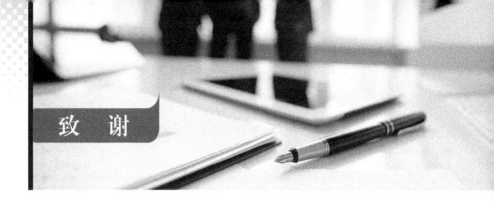

致 谢

本书的撰写中还参考了以下文献，特此感谢！

[1] Kliewer M A. Writing it up：a step-by-step guide to publication for beginning investigators[J]. J Nucl Med Technol,2006, 34(1):53－59.

[2] Balch C M, McMasters K M, Klimberg V S, et al. Steps to getting your manuscript published in a high-quality medical journal[J]. Ann Surg Oncol,2018,25(4):850－855.

[3] Barroga E, Matanguihan G J. Creating logical flow when writing scientific articles[J]. J Korean Med Sci, 2021, 36(40):e275.

[4] Kojima T, Popiel H A. Proper scholarly writing for non-native English-speaking authors：choosing active and passive voice, rewording, and refining texts[J]. J Korean Med Sci,2022, 37(44):e312.

[5] Kojima T, Popiel H A. Using guidelines to improve scientific writing：tips on use of correct verb tenses for non-native English-speaking researchers [J]. J Korean Med Sci, 2022, 37(29):e226.

[6] Yakhontova T. What nonnative authors should know when writing research articles in English[J]. J Korean Med Sci, 2021,36(35):e237.

[7] Citations [EB/OL]. https://www. biomedcentral. com/ getpublished/editorial-policies♯Citations.

[8] APA. Write With Clarity, Precision, and Inclusion[EB/ OL]. https://apastyle. apa. org.